MW00844516

Oncoplastic and Reconstructive Surgery for Breast Cancer

A. Fitoussi · MG Berry
B. Couturaud · R. J. Salmon

Oncoplastic and Reconstructive Surgery for Breast Cancer

The Institut Curie Experience

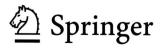

Editors

A. Fitoussi
Institut Curie
26 rue d'Ulm
Paris 70005
France

B. Couturaud
Institut Curie
26 rue d'Ulm
Paris 75005
France

MG Berry
Institut Curie
26 rue d'Ulm
Paris 75005
France

R. J. Salmon
Institut Curie
26 rue d'Ulm
Paris 75005
France

Acknowledgements: Doctors K. B. Clough, C. Nos, H. Charitansky, V. Forchotte, S. Alran, A. G. Pollet and the surgeons of the Institut Curie Breast Study Group. S Perdereau for technical assistance. The authors are particularly indebted to Y. Kirova and A. Fourquet (Radiotherapy), J-Y. Pierga (Medical Oncology), S. Dolbeaut and A. Brédart (Onco-psychology) and D Stoppa-Lyonnet and P This (Genetics) for the relevant chapters.

Originally published: A. Fitoussi, B. Couturaud, R.J. Salmon: Chirurgie oncoplastique et reconstruction dans le cancer du sein. Techniques et indications.
© Springer-Verlag, France, Paris 2008

ISBN 978-3-642-00143-7   ISBN 978-3-642-00144-4 (eBook)
DOI 10.1007/978-3-642-00144-4
Springer Dordrecht Heidelberg London New York

Library of Congress Control Number: 2009944021

© Springer-Verlag Berlin Heidelberg 2009
This work is subject to copyright. All rights are reserved, whether the whole or part of the material is concerned, specifically the rights of translation, reprinting, reuse of illustrations, recitation, broadcasting, reproduction on microfilm or in any other way, and storage in data banks. Duplication of this publication or parts thereof is permitted only under the provisions of the German Copyright Law of September 9, 1965, in its current version, and permission for use must always be obtained from Springer. Violations are liable to prosecution under the German Copyright Law.
The use of general descriptive names, registered names, trademarks, etc. in this publication does not imply, even in the absence of a specific statement, that such names are exempt from the relevant protective laws and regulations and therefore free for general use.
Product liability: The publishers cannot guarantee the accuracy of any information about dosage and application contained in this book. In every individual case the user must check such information by consulting the relevant literature.

Cover design: Frido Steinen-Broo, eStudio Calamar, Spain.

Printed on acid-free paper

Springer is part of Springer Science+Business Media (www.springer.com)

Preface

Whilst contemporary breast cancer management is multidisciplinary, the surgeon continues to play a key role, particularly as the irradiation mandated by breast-conserving therapy only worsens suboptimal results. Today's patients are ever less accepting of poor aesthetic outcomes, and oncoplastic breast surgery (OBS) was derived directly from cosmetic surgery for this very reason.

This book is aimed at the practising breast surgeon, of any grade, who may be unfamiliar with the full range of techniques available for the management of breast cancer, particularly in such a rapidly evolving subspecialty as OBS. It will also be of interest to anyone involved in the care of breast cancer patients, and with that in mind employs a minimum of text, and is supported by the results of systematic evaluations performed at a centre that pioneered OBS in the late 1980s. The Institut Curie has continued to develop and refine the techniques in order to create a practical system with which any breast cancer can be approached.

It is richly illustrated with clinical examples of the numerous surgeons who have passed through the Breast Study Group at the Institut Curie, and we hope other surgeons will be able to incorporate these techniques into their clinical practice and produce patients as satisfied as our own.

Contents

Introduction

Breast cancer is a growing public health problem in many countries: in France, 42,000 new cases were diagnosed in 2006, which corresponds to an incidence of one in ten women. Fortunately, this cancer can be diagnosed at an increasingly early stage. In 1980, 15% of cancers were diagnosed at stage T0–1. This rate has since increased to more than 50%, and obviously the smaller the cancer the easier disease control becomes. Early mammographic screening detection as a result of individual strategies and more recently in national campaigns, along with readily available information and general quality of life improvements, have all played a role in this evolution. However, the reason for the paradoxical increase in the incidence of breast cancer and its diagnosis at an earlier stage currently remains unclear. Nutritional and hormonal factors may be important, but such studies are complex; their results require long surveillance periods, and individual behaviour is difficult to modify.

As a consequence of the earlier diagnosis of breast cancer, aesthetic outcomes are becoming ever more important and, even if this has not yet become a legal requirement, our patients are legitimately ever more demanding in this regard. The validity of "conservative treatment" for small tumours is beyond question, but it is equally important that the treatment should yield results that are "cosmetic" in quality. Of course, tumour size, tumour-to-breast volume ratio, location within the breast, proximity to the areola or infra-mammary fold, tissue quality and comorbidities are important contributors to the aesthetic outcome. Additionally, adjuvant treatments, radiotherapy and chemotherapy, play a vital role in the ultimate aesthetic result. It must also be borne in mind that a poor initial surgical result is usually only worsened by subsequent treatments.

The "breast" surgeon must therefore anticipate the quality of his results in combination with his knowledge of other treatments and their effects on both scars and breast volume.

The contribution of plastic surgery techniques to breast cancer has given birth to what is now referred to as "oncoplastic breast surgery" (OBS). For a while, this was reserved for the prevention of poor results in cancers of the lower pole, and involved performing a bilateral breast reduction in those patients with breasts that had an appropriate volume. Similar techniques have subsequently been adapted for other locations, as will be discussed.

There are, however, a number of situations where mastectomy is required, including recurrence after conservative treatment, multicentric or multifocal cancer, genetic predisposition to BRCA1/2 mutation (whether identified or not), and occasionally by specific request of the patient. In these cases, breast reconstruction may be discussed and should be proposed as part of the treatment strategy. If, as is standard, one avoids suggesting reconstruction to a patient who may receive irradiation to the thoracic wall, a number of other situations present themselves and should be discussed within the multidisciplinary team (MDT) setting, in addition to with the patient herself. It should always be remembered that the priority remains treatment of the cancer, and that aesthetics should never result in inadequate or incomplete oncological gestures. It is also true that in certain cases these dual targets (oncological and aesthetic) may be contradictory, which is why it is important that such surgery is undertaken either by surgeons familiar with this type of management or by two teams that combine the dual competencies. It is, therefore, fundamentally a type of multidisciplinarity in which the well informed patient's opinion is

A. Fitoussi et al., *Oncoplastic and Reconstructive Surgery for Breast Cancer*,
DOI: 10.1007/978-3-642-00144-4, © Springer-Verlag Berlin Heidelberg 2009

essential. Remember also that aesthetics was a philosophy before becoming a branch of surgery.

The problems that our patients encounter during the course of their cancer management are not always related to the size of their scars, and it is an illusion to think that merely conserving an acceptable form and good quality scars will erase the trauma that they experience both during treatment and in subsequent years. It involves nothing less than taking charge of their entire body image, as a function of their age, and trying to simplify their personal life and relations in order to enable them to rebuild their life more easily.

This work is the result of a revolution in breast cancer care that has taken place over more than 30 years. All of the surgeons who have passed through the Institut Curie have contributed in some way to this evolution through reflection, analysis of results, and through papers and presentations at national and international meetings. It is obvious to all of the surgeons at the Institut that this is the work of a team, a team whose members have changed throughout the years, but a team that has always prioritised caring for the sick and advancing the quality of care.

Anatomical Review

The mammary gland is situated on the anterior thorax and is by definition bilateral and symmetrical. Its form, volume and contents vary with age, making precise characterisation impossible. Glorified by artists throughout the ages, the breast occupies an important place in the image of women in our culture, and in its beauty rests a fundamental element of femininity. This beauty is, however, both subjective and determined by an anatomy and physiology that will not be described in extensive detail here.

The breast is primarily a secretory gland, comprising lobules that produce milk for lactation and ducts that run from the lobules towards the areola and nipple. It is at the lobulo-ductal junction that breast cancers develop; these can be differentiated predominantly into ductal or lobular subtypes. The genesis of these cancers remains imprecisely understood, and what makes some become ductal whilst others become lobular is also a mystery.

The mammary gland is attached to the surrounding skin by a fibrous tissue known as the "crests of Duret". The gland itself is surrounded by connective tissue that varies in density with age. Breast density is one of the factors that affect the interpretation of screening mammography; in fact, it is one of the criteria for mammographic assessment. One can generalise that the younger a patient, the more dense the breast and thus the more difficult the mammographic analysis. The breast is attached to the pectoralis major muscle fascia via fibrous tissue that is resiliant but allows the gland a degree of mobility with respect to the muscle.

The gland's lymphatic drainage occurs through channels that head towards a periareolar circle. Two principal and two variable accessory channels arise from this periareolar circle; these lead mainly towards the anterolateral thoracic group of the axilla, in contact with the serratus anterior muscle (where the sentinel node is usually located). There are further channels of smaller calibre and variable position that drain into the internal mammary, supraclavicular, and—on occasion—transpectorally towards Rotter's nodes. This drainage pattern was first described in 1874 by the French anatomist Sappey (Fig. 1). It was rediscovered a century later in vivo as an advantageous by-product of sentinel lymph node biopsy (SLNB). Overall, the lymphatic drainage of the breast occurs predominantly towards the axilla.

Anatomically, the axilla is a crude pyramid, the boundaries (Fig. 2) of which are:

- The serratus anterior muscle medially, on which lies the long thoracic nerve
- The pectoralis major and minor muscles anteriorly
- The tendon of the long head of biceps in front of the teres major, with the subscapular and latissimus dorsi muscles posterolaterally
- The axillary vein, as the apex

The base of the axilla comprises the clavipectoro-axillary fascia, which is of variable thickness. It inserts superiorly into the clavicle and subscapular muscle but is lost in the inferior axilla and forms part of the suspensory ligament of the axilla. At times a nightmare for anatomists and trainee surgeons alike, it is nevertheless the key to axillary surgery (Fig. 3).

Once this fascia is opened, accessing the principal neurovascular structures becomes a simple task, with the cavity being essentially filled with fat. The opened axilla allows dissection of its contents, and identification of the fascia also allows for its closure, thus avoiding the need to insert a drain after axillary clearance.

The axillary nodes are distributed anatomically into five groups; however, since the work of Berg three levels have been recognised. These levels are defined by their relationship to the pectoralis minor

A. Fitoussi et al., *Oncoplastic and Reconstructive Surgery for Breast Cancer,*
DOI: 10.1007/978-3-642-00144-4, © Springer-Verlag Berlin Heidelberg 2009

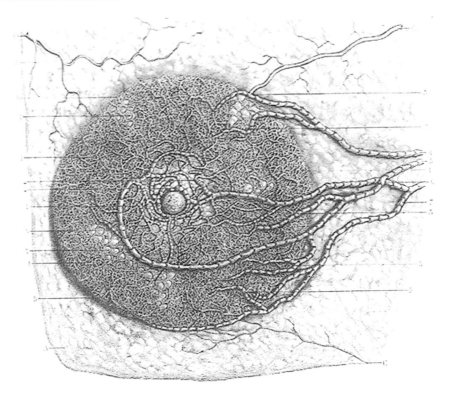

Fig. 1 Plate from Sappey's treatise showing the lymphatic drainage of the breast, which is predominantly to the axilla

tendon: the first lying inferior, the second posterior, and the third superior (Fig. 4).

This distinction is somewhat artificial, in part due to anatomical variations of the muscle, which are numerous, and in part because the fat and nodes exist in a continuum rather than in discrete groups. Magnetic resonance imaging (MRI) has also confirmed the considerable variability with upper limb movement, a fact that underlines the inherent difficulties in determining correct radiation doses to this region.

Custom has it that classical dissection comprises only the removal of the first two of Berg's levels and stops inferior to the axillary vein. This allows the brachial nodes to be avoided, since damage to these predisposes to lymphoedema of the arm following dissection.

Posteriorly, the neurovascular pedicle of latissimus dorsi must be preserved during dissection. The external mammary vein, however, may be sacrificed and the second perforating intercostal nerve can either be preserved or not according to preference. The latter provides sensation to the medial surface of the upper arm and posterior shoulder and its section produces a characteristic dysaesthesia that disappears within a year.

Knowledge of the boundaries of the axilla allows dissection without any difficulty. Since the introduction

of SLNB, the sentinel node(s) can be identified easily without requiring formal identification of the axillary walls. The technique of colourimetry and/or isotopic detection can mark where the node lies in the axillary fat, but it is essential to have opened the fascia to allow access to it. This is why retractile scarring of the fascia makes dissection difficult when reoperating on the axilla.

It became apparent that axillary dissection resulted in lymphocoeles in more than 60% of cases, necessitating suction drainage with occasionally repeated percutaneous drainage. The aetiology of these collections remains unknown, and preventative measures seem to have little efficacy. During drainage, it is important to avoid infecting the lymphocoele, particularly when a prosthesis has been inserted.

Anatomical Position of the Breast

The breast comprises four arbitrarily defined segments (Fig. 5):

- Segment I corresponds to the anterior thoracic portion between the clavicle and the supramammary fold

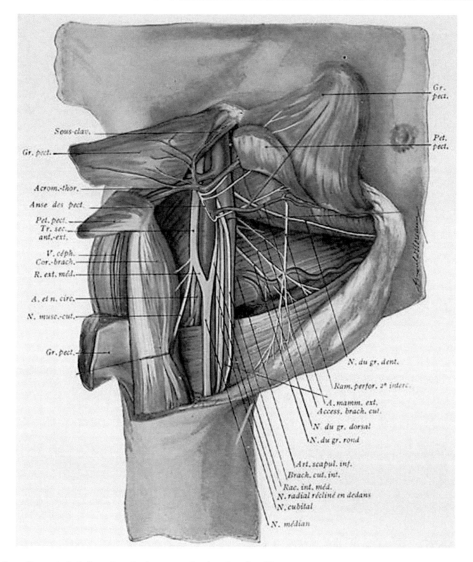

Fig. 2 Plate from Beau et al. delineating the important landmarks of axillary anatomy

- Segment II between the supramammary fold and the upper border of the areola
- The nipple–areolar complex (NAC)
- Segment III from the inferior areolar border to the inframammary fold
- Segment IV is the thoracic skin between the inframammary fold and the costal margin

The principal dimensions of the breast are (Fig. 6):

- Segments I + II together are of the order of 15–17 cm
- The NAC is 4–5 cm
- Segment III is 4–6 cm

- The distance separating the midline and medial areolar border is 9–11 cm

The mammary height is defined by the lengths of segments II, III and the NAC.

The standard anatomical proportions of the breast are as follows:

- Height/projection: > 2
- Height/width: 0.7–1.3

The breast is located between the third and seventh ribs.

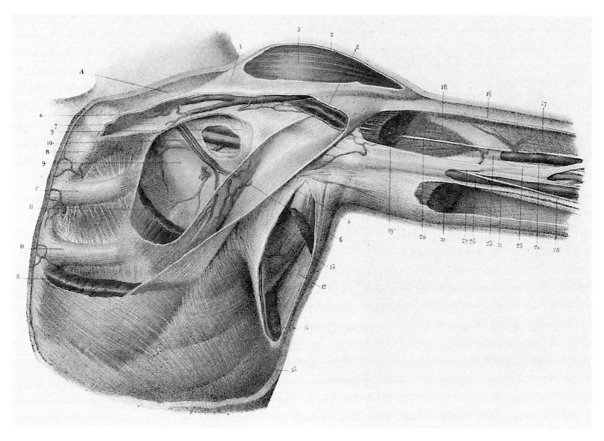

Fig. 3 Beau et al's detailed representation of the intricate interconnections of the clavipectoro-axillary fascia

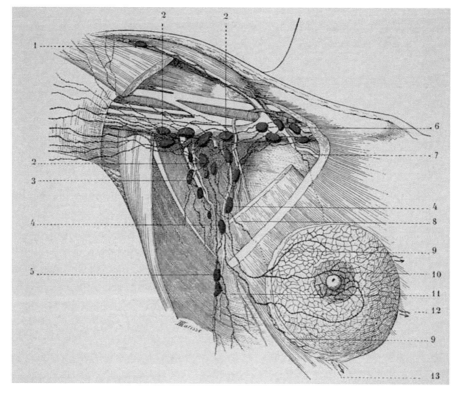

Fig. 4 Axillary lymphatic anatomy according to Sappey with reference to Berg's levels for axillary dissection

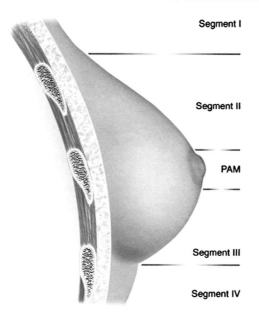

Fig. 5 Segments of the female breast—lateral view

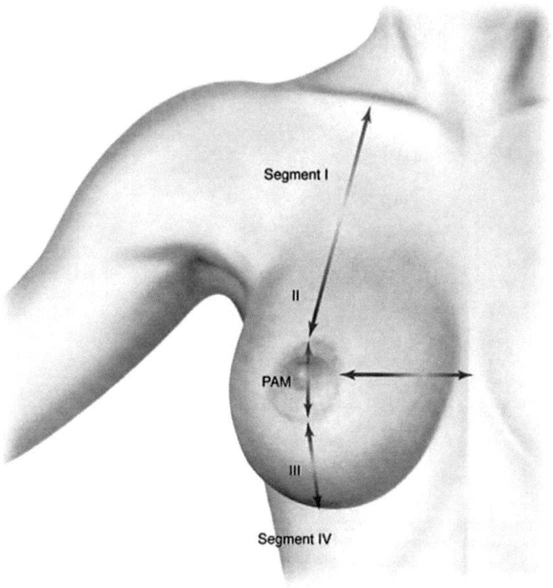

Fig. 6 Segments of the female breast—anteroposterior view

References

Bonamy C, Broca P, Beau E (1867) Atlas d' anatomic du corps humain. Masson, Paris

Sappey C (1874) Anatomie, physiologie, pathologie des vaisseaux lymphatiques. Adrien Delahaye Libraire Editeur, Paris

Berg JW (1955) The significance of axillary node levels in the study of breast carcinoma. Cancer 8:776–778

Incisions for Tumours Not Requiring Oncoplastic Surgery

Conservative Treatment

This chapter is concerned with "simple" tumourectomies; that is, those with a tumour-to-breast volume proportion and location that permit wide excision in a conservative fashion without the need for an oncoplastic technique.

Basic Principles of Incisions

One must always design the incisions with a marker prior to surgical intervention in both the sitting and standing positions, placing them within the boundaries of a future mastectomy wherever possible.

Except when skin excision is required, direct incisions should be avoided in the inferior quadrants, the décolletage and near the sternum, which has a high rate of hypertrophic and even keloid scarring.

Avoid curvilinear incisions in the inferior and superolateral quadrants and radial incisions close to the areola, which are the source of nipple retraction.

A periareolar incision may involve one half of the areolar circumference if necessary. A medial or lateral extension can be added in the case of a small areola. Alternatively, a combined radial and periareolar incision will not produce areolar retraction.

One must always repair the parenchymal defect to avoid unsightly distortions.

Wide Local Excisions

Also referred to as tumourectomies or partial mastectomies, these aim at adequate oncological surgery that is also aesthetic.

Wide Local Excisions Without Skin Excision

These involve tumours that have not produced skin retraction.

The skin is first dissected from the gland widely enough to facilitate remodelling without any distortion of the skin.

Tumour resection extends from the skin to the prepectoral fascia as a fusiform excision, the long axis of which corresponds to a ray of the breast (Fig. 1.1a). It passes at least 1 cm macroscopically outside the tumour and is guided by bidigital palpation: simultaneously beneath the skin and the deep surface of the gland. The remainder of the gland is also palpated bidigitally.

Metal clips are placed on the perimysium and at the tumour excision margins, and also to orientate the specimen clearly for histopathological examination. Subsequent re-excisions are similarly orientated.

The gland is usually raised from the muscle plane to facilitate rotation or advancement of glandular flaps, which reconstitute the defect left by tumourectomy (Figs. 1.1b and 1.1c). Glandular repair utilises absorbable sutures and the full depth must be apposed to avoid a cutaneous dimple. If such dimpling results from gland remodelling, the skin is simply dissected in these areas. Drains, suction or otherwise, are not routinely used.

A. Fitoussi et al., *Oncoplastic and Reconstructive Surgery for Breast Cancer,*
DOI: 10.1007/978-3-642-00144-4_1, © Springer-Verlag Berlin Heidelberg 2009

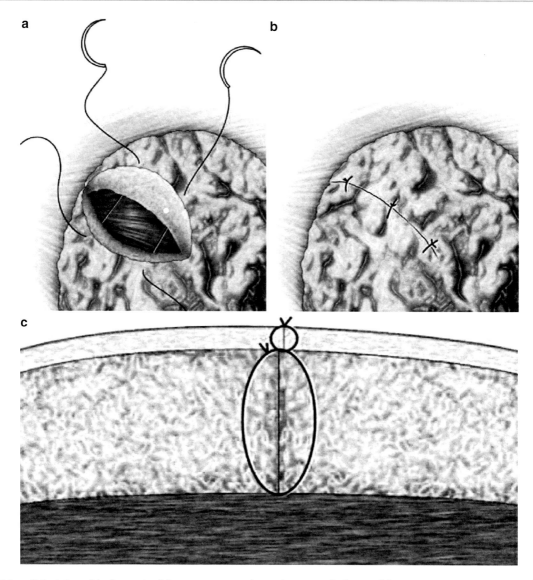

Fig. 1.1 **a** Orientation of the long axis of the tumourectomy along a breast ray; **b** closure of the tumourectomy; **c** transverse view of layered tumourectomy closure with dead-space obliteration

Superior Quadrant Tumours

Treatment of these tumours depends on the quadrant and the distance from the NAC. They may require an oncoplastic approach by an omega or lateral mammaplasty (see Chap. 2).

If the tumour is close to the areola, a periareolar incision is preferred, perhaps with a radial extension for small areolae.

For the superolateral quadrant, a direct radial incision may be used when the tumour is too far from either the axilla or areola. For those close to the axilla, breast and axillary surgery is often possible through the same incision, which starts in the axilla and extends radially towards the nipple. Raising skin from the gland prevents the incision on the breast from being too long. En bloc excision of gland and axillary contents is then possible as a fusiform, enabling direct glandular repair as described above (Fig. 1.2).

For tumours close to the lateral mammary fold (LMF) beneath the axilla, we favour a vertical axillary incision (along the palpable lateral border of pectoralis major muscle) that can be extended into the LMF.

Both types of incision may be applied for SLNB, in which case the node(s) is harvested before the mammary

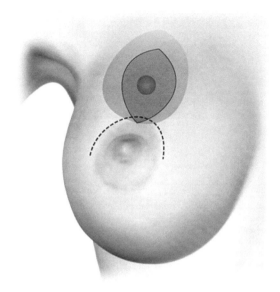

Fig. 1.2 Semielliptical tumourectomy along a breast ray accessed through a periareolar skin incision

incision and sent for frozen section analysis. Drain insertion is not routine.

For tumours at the junction of the superior quadrants, far from the areola, a direct curvilinear incision is suggested.

For tumours of the superomedial quadrant and remote from the areola, one may use a direct radial incision in the natural breast creases in order to avoid incisions in the décolletage.

For tumours at the medial quadrant junction, a radial incision may be required if distant from the areola, although sternal incisions must be avoided. The same radial approach is applicable for peripheral lateral quadrant tumours.

Tumours of the Inferior Quadrants

Direct incisions are to be avoided because they produce cutaneoglandular retraction with aesthetic sequelae that alter the form and projection of the gland. A radial incision in the inferior quadrants results in more areolar retraction than a periareolar incision and the aesthetic consequences can be significant.

Oncoplastic techniques are generally required in small-volume glands in the inferior quadrants, particularly inferomedially.

For tumours close to the areola, one should use a periareolar incision.

For tumours at the junction of the inferior quadrants distant from the areola, a straight vertical incision may be selected with gland excision along a vertical axis (the only situation where a radial incision is possible in the inferior quadrants).

For tumours close to the IMF, an incision just above the fold is preferred.

Wide Local Excision Requiring Skin Resection

This technique is used for tumours close to the skin, generally with retraction. Those actually involving the skin (T4b) are not typically an indication for conservative treatment.

A direct excision with skin sacrifice may be required in any quadrant. A semielliptical skin excision is used for radial incisions. A "croissant" excision is preferred for curvilinear incisions.

A radial incision is preferred in the superolateral, superomedial, lateral and inferior quadrants. An oncoplastic technique is preferred in the inferior quadrants. Curvilinear incision is reserved for tumours at the superior quadrant junction. At the junction of the medial quadrants, both types of incision are possible in the context of skin excision.

For central tumours close to the NAC, its excision is indicated (see Chap. 2).

Axillary Incisions

At the Institute Curie, a transverse axillary incision is the rule for either SLNB or axillary dissection.

Axillary Dissection

The incision is transverse, horizontal and gently curved in an axillary crease two fingers' breadth from the axillary apex. It does not pass beyond the borders of pectoralis major anteriorly and latissimus dorsi posteriorly. This incision allows for a direct approach to the axilla, after opening the clavipectoro-axillary fascia, with full dissection of the adipocellular axillary

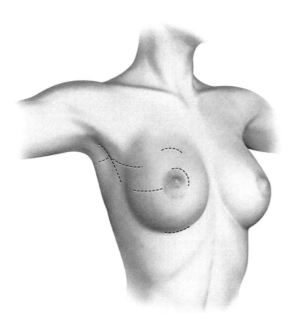

Fig. 1.3 Incisions of choice for breast and axillary access

contents. This incision is less likely to produce retractile axillary scars and is highly aesthetic. It may be extended onto the breast in a radial direction towards the nipple for tumours of the superolateral quadrant (Fig. 1.3). Axillary dissection is performed according to the standard anatomical boundaries.

Drainage

In our institution, a size 10 Fr suction drain is usually placed, but dead space closure is an option. It remains in place until 50 ml or less has drained, and is removed within seven days. The debate over drainage—whether and for how long it is needed, or whether to use dead-space closure—remains open for discussion.

Sentinel Node Biopsy

The incision is placed transversely in an axillary crease. It is small (2 cm) and extended only for dissection. The clavipectoro-axillary fascia is opened, and the node(s) identified and harvested. Here too the dead space may be closed.

Nonconservative Treatment

Mastectomy

The radical mastectomy typically performed in our unit is that modified by Madden et al. (1972). It comprises complete extirpation of the mammary gland along with axillary dissection of Berg levels 1 and 2 in an en bloc fashion. Resection of the muscles, pectoralis major or minor, three-level dissection (Halsted 1882) (Halsted 1907), or mastectomy associated with pectoralis minor resection and three-level dissection (Patey and Dyson 1948) are no longer performed.

In extensive ductal carcinoma in situ (DCIS), mastectomy can be performed with a low dissection guided by blue-dyed sentinel nodes.

The incision is the same whether or not there is associated axillary surgery, and it must allow the excision of both the NAC and the tumour(s).

Generally, a horizontal or oblique incision is made along the axis of a line from the axilla to the xiphoid. Occasionally, with unusually located tumours, atypical incisions are required, and scars from a previous tumourectomy should be incorporated.

The amount of skin excision must allow tension-free closure, but must also be sufficiently wide to prevent a lateral "dog ear".

For the horizontal incision, the axis lies at the midlevel of the thorax and the excision is semielliptical.

In the oblique incision, the axis passes from the xiphoid to the axilla, and this scar has the advantage of being less visible in the décolletage.

For upper extremity tumours, far from the nipple, the incision may be in the form of a boomerang, with one point incorporating the tumour and heading vertically to 12 o'clock, and the other heading perpendicularly laterally. The nipple is thus located at the angle of the boomerang. This scar allows for easy access to the axilla, removes the tumour and nipple, and respects the cleavage (Fig. 1.4).

For superomedial or inferolateral tumours remote from the nipple, we suggest an oblique incision perpendicular to the usual axis (Fig. 1.5).

For inferior quadrant tumours close to the IMF, we suggest either a low horizontal excision removing the IMF and NAC or one in the shape of an anchor

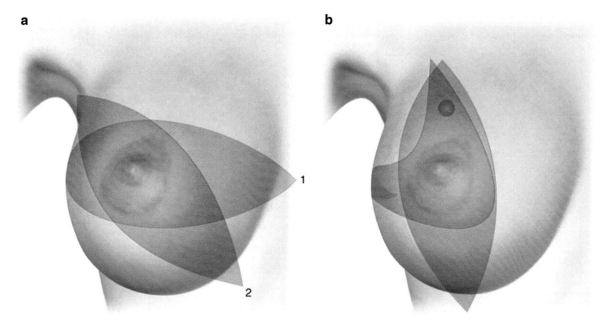

Fig. 1.4 **a** Horizontal/oblique mastectomy incisions; **b** vertical/boomerang incisions for mastectomy

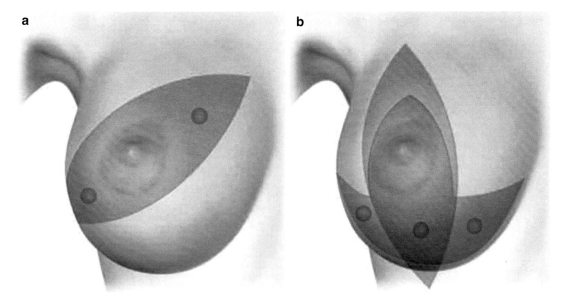

Fig. 1.5 **a** reverse oblique mastectomy incision for tumours of the superomedial and inferolateral quadrants; **b** use of the inverted-T mastectomy excision

(inverted-T) with a horizontal base and an inferior line situated below the IMF. The NAC is included within the anchor, which points to 12 o'clock (Fig. 1.5).

Drainage

Two suction drains are placed in mastectomies with axillary dissection: one in the mastectomy bed, the other in the axilla. We do not generally close the axillary dead space in this situation.

Sentinel Nodes

Breast-conserving surgery and node excision has been the treatment of choice in the majority of patients with early (T1N0 or N1a) stage breast cancer since 2000.

A history of previous plastic surgery may affect the lymphatic network, notably with periareolar incisions, and so oncological surgeons must be careful when using SLNB in such cases.

Studies reporting SLNB after previous plastic surgery are rare and comprise three types:

– History of bilateral breast augmentation and SLNB feasibility
– Influence of the axillary route for implant placement on lymphatic drainage
– History of tumourectomy in SLNB identification

There are no published studies, at the time of writing, on breast reduction, particularly in relation to periareolar scars, NAC repositioning and SLNB.

After Previous Plastic or Breast Surgery

History of Augmentation and Feasibility of SLNB

Gray et al. (2004) reported a retrospective review of patients that had undergone bilateral breast augmentation managed with breast-conserving surgery or SLNB at the Mayo Clinic. Among the 39 patients studied, 11

underwent lymphoscintigraphy with sentinel node excision: each lymphoscintigram showed at least one node. The identification rate was 100% and the mean number of sentinel nodes identified was 2.5 (range 1–4). Nine patients (81.8%) underwent dissection to the axillary vein in order to evaluate the false-negative rate. Two patients without dissection had in situ cancer or microcalcifications only. The false-negative rate was 0%. For the two without dissection, no evidence of recurrence was seen at 20 and 24 months of follow up.

Influence on Lymphatic Drainage of the Axillary Route for Implant Insertion

A Brazilian study from H Sao Paulo contributed 36 patients (Munhoz et al. 2007).

This anatomical study of lymphatic drainage by lymphoscintigraphy involved patients who had previous plastic surgery (implant insertion via an axillary incision). There were no SLNBs, but all had a lymphoscintigram one week before and ten days after the intervention. Preoperative scintigraphy identified a mean of two sentinel nodes on the left and right sides. There was a failure to identify sentinel nodes at ten days in two patients (7.6%). These initial results show that sentinel node detection is possible in cases of axillary incision in the majority of patients.

Prior Tumourectomy in Sentinel Node Identification and False-Negative Rate

Two North American teams have published their results in previous tumourectomy (Table 1.1). The diagnosis was frequently made by biopsy before axillary surgery.

In these two series—one retrospective (Haigh et al. 2000) the other prospective (Wong et al. 2002)—patients with T1–2 N0 breast cancers had a preliminary diagnostic or percutaneous biopsy, followed by axillary (SLNB or dissection) with or without breast surgery. There was no significant difference in the rate of identification and false negatives between the two groups (Table 1.1).

Table 1.1 Results of previous tumourectomy. From studies performed by Haigh and Wong

	Haigh et al. (2000)		Wong et al. (2002)	
	$n = 181$ (surgical excision)	$n = 130$ (percutaneous biopsy)	$n = 763$ (surgical excision)	$n = 1,443$ (percutaneous biopsy)
Rate of sentinel node identification (%)	83	77	92.8	92.4
False negative rate (%)	3.2	0	8.3	7.9

Previous Breast Reduction Associated with Periareolar Incisions and NAC Repositioning

There are no published articles that investigate sentinel node identification following periareolar surgery. In his anatomical treatise, Sappey (1874) demonstrated that all breast lymphatics led to the nipple and formed an areolar plexus. Two main lymphatic channels arise from this plexus, one draining laterally to the axilla and the other medially, which form an organised subareolar circle that then heads towards the axilla. One can imagine division of these channels by previous surgery and consequent modifications of lymph flow that may be documented lymphographically (Salmon et al. 2007).

SLNB During an Oncoplastic Procedure

The indications are the same as those for breast-conserving treatment (i.e. T1N0 or N1a tumours).

The process of searching for and excising the sentinel node(s) is essentially identical to that described previously.

Initial access to the axilla can be achieved through a short axillary incision (independent of the oncoplastic incision), particularly in surgery of the inferior quadrants, or can be combined with oncoplastic incisions, notably in the lateral or superior quadrants.

References

Gray RJ, Forstner-Barthell AW, Pockaj B, et al. (2004) Breast-conserving therapy and sentinel lymph node biopsy are feasible in cancer patients with previous implant breast augmentation. Am J Surg 188:122–5

Haigh P, Hansen N, Qi K, et al. (2000) Biopsy method and excision volume do not affect success rate of subsequent sentinel lymph node dissection in breast cancer. Ann Surg Oncol 7:21–7

Halsted WS (1907) The result of radical operations for the cure of carcinoma of the breast. Ann Surg 146(1):1–19

Madden JL, Kandalaft S, Bourque RA (1972) Modified radical mastectomy. Ann Surg 175(5):624–34

Munhoz AM, Aldrighi C, Ono C, et al. (2007) The influence of sub-fascial transaxillary breast augmentation in axillary lymphatic drainage patterns and sentinel lymph node detection. Ann Plast Surg 58:141–9

Patey DH, Dyson WH (1948) Prognosis of carcinoma of breast in relation to type of operation performed. Br J Cancer 2:7–13

Salmon RJ, Montemagno S, Laki F, et al. (2007) Réseaux lymphatiques de la glande mammaire: 1—identification du ganglion sentinelle revue à la lumière des anciens anatomistes. J Chir (Paris) 144:72–4

Sappey C (1874) Anatomie, physiologie, pathologie des vaisseaux lymphatiques. Adrien Delahaye Librairie Éditeur, Paris

Wong SL, Edwards M, Chao C, et al. (2002) The effect of prior breast biopsy method and concurrent definitive breast procedure on success and accuracy of sentinel lymph node biopsy. Ann Surg Oncol 9:272–7

Breast-Conserving Surgery for Central Tumours: "NACectomies"

Introduction

Centrally located tumours have long been considered to be more serious, multifocal and more likely to recur. In fact, this is not the case; the only real problem is ensuring that the breast is preserved with a "normal" form following breast-conserving surgery and adjuvant radiotherapy.

As with more peripheral tumours, central tumours may also benefit from breast-conserving surgery.

Several techniques have been used depending on the tumour and the size and form of the breast.

Periareolar Technique

This comprises an en bloc excision, via a periareolar incision, of the nipple-areola complex (NAC) and underlying tissue as far as the prepectoral fascia (Fig. 2.1). The mammary gland is then raised at this plane and reconstitution of the gland effected by approximating the breast parenchyma. This is performed from deep to superficial, and produces a breast with a reduced base width but increased projection. In this way, one can avoid the "flat" appearance seen in the reconstructed breast following central tumourectomy without gland remodelling (Fig. 2.2). A submammary drain is used and, where required, the skin is raised separately to facilitate closure in a "purse-string" fashion (Fig. 2.3).

Horizontal Technique

This is similar to the periareolar technique in all respects except the skin incision, which is semielliptical, in the shape of an eye, with the NAC resembling the iris (Fig. 2.4 and plate 2.1). Gland remodelling is identical, but skin closure is direct, yielding a transverse linear scar (Fig. 2.5). In cases of more pronounced ptosis, a longer incision may be used. This technique thus approximates the omega mammaplasty without NAC preservation.

Mammaplasty-Associated Techniques

If the tumour is larger or deeper, and the breast parenchymal volume allows a breast reduction can be performed in association with NACectomy. The design is generally either purely vertical or an inverted T (Fig. 2.5 and plate 2.2), but it can also involve other plasties, such as J-plasty or lateral mammaplasty.

A symmetrising procedure on the contralateral breast is frequently required in a subsequent operation after adjuvant radiotherapy has been completed. All techniques are available, depending on the requirements: periareolar is usually used for small modifications, but vertical-scar, inverted-T and lateral mammaplasty are also used according to the final form of the treated breast. NAC reconstruction is conveniently performed at this second sitting, with either areolar skin grafting and a nipple graft or local flaps (Little's technique), or areolar tattooing and local flaps (F flap) (see Chap. 6).

A. Fitoussi et al., *Oncoplastic and Reconstructive Surgery for Breast Cancer,*
DOI: 10.1007/978-3-642-00144-4_2, © Springer-Verlag Berlin Heidelberg 2009

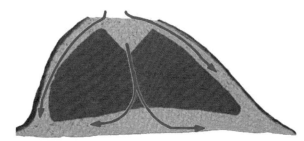

Fig. 2.1 Dissection planes for tumourectomy

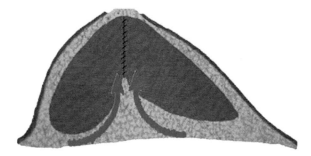

Fig. 2.2 Parenchymal flaps allowing filling of the tumourectomy defect and reconstitution of the breast mound

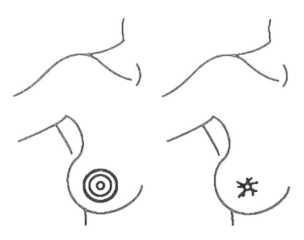

Fig. 2.3 NACectomy with purse-string closure

Discussion

Central tumours represent 5–20% of breast cancers and are treated in the same fashion as those that are more peripherally located. Resection must be similarly wide to avoid surgical re-excisions and secondary mastectomies.

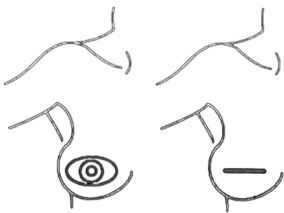

Fig. 2.4 NACectomy with short transverse scar

Overall survival, risk of recurrence and metastatic disease are identical to other tumour locations.

Deep central tumours that are more than 3 cm from the areola are considered to be "peripheral" and are therefore treated accordingly.

In a series of 146 patients at the Institut Curie, central tumours represented 7.5% of the cases, had a mean size of 21.5 mm, and a mean distance from the areola of 5.2 mm. The most common techniques were horizontal ($n = 72\%$), periareolar ($n = 14\%$) and inverted T ($n = 6\%$). In the remainder ($n = 9\%$), other techniques such as lateral and vertical-scar mammaplasty were employed.

Symmetrising surgery was undertaken at the same time in only 17%.

The complication rate was low, of the order of 9%, comprising predominantly haematomas, wound breakdown, delayed healing and infection.

Histopathological evaluation showed:

– Clear excision margins in more than 80%
– Minimally clear margins (within 2 mm) in 11%
– Involved margins in 9%
– Areolar invasion/involvement in 62%

These incomplete margins were treated with:

– Completion mastectomy in 9 patients
– A further wide excision plus radiotherapy in 2 patients
– An additional "boost" of local radiotherapy in 12 patients

Secondary NAC reconstruction was performed in a third of patients.

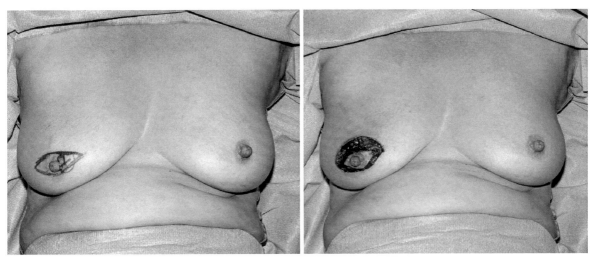

a medial retroareolar tumour   b horizontal semielliptical excision with skin-gland dissection

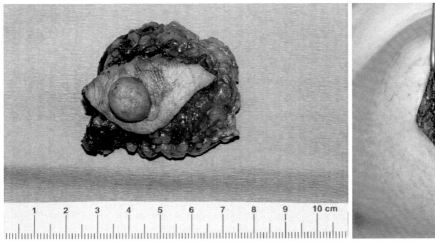

c operative specimen with nipple areolar complex en bloc with the
glandular cone

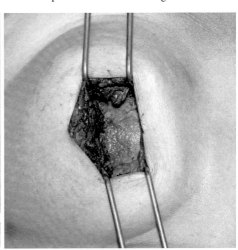

d NACectomy to the prepectoral fascia

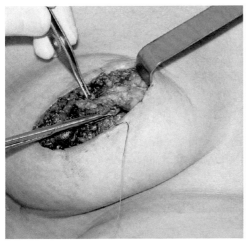

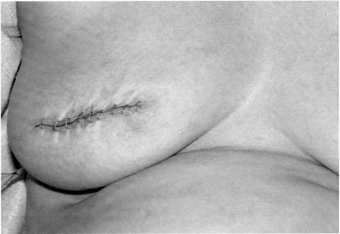

e reconstitution of glandular cone by approximation
commencing deeply

f skin closure giving a good result in both form and volume

Plate 2.1a–f Surgical treatment of central tumours; NACectomy with horizontal incision

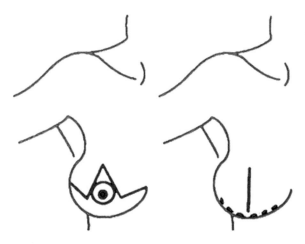

Fig. 2.5 NACectomy with inverted-T scar

Patients were satisfied in more than 90% of cases, with a failure and poor result rate of 4.3%.

With a mean follow up in excess of 64 months, the overall survival was 96%, disease-free survival was 91%, and five-year local recurrence rate was 8.2%, half of which were remote from the initial tumourectomy.

Conclusion

The management of central, retroareolar tumours is comparable to that of other conservative treatments. The challenge is to remodel the breast such that it retains a normal form prior to radiotherapy, because this form becomes fixed and subsequent surgery on an irradiated breast is much more difficult. The quality of the initial result from primary surgery is therefore paramount. (Results are displayed in Plates 2.3 and 2.4).

Plastic Surgical Techniques in Breast Cancer Surgery (Oncoplastic Breast Surgery)

Introduction

Conservative surgery in breast cancer management has long been the standard for tumours < 3 cm. More recent series have extended the indications for breast-

conserving surgery to include tumour sizes of up to 4 cm (Fisher et al. 1995), 5 cm (van Dongen 2000; Jacobson et al. 1995), and even larger for intraductal cancer (Fisher et al. 1995; Solin et al. 1996).

The predominant issue remains the compromise between a wide excision with clear margins and a satisfactory aesthetic result. This problem is far easier to solve if the breast volume is sufficient to allow an oncoplastic technique.

Thanks to a variety of plastic surgical techniques, this conflict can now be resolved in the majority of cases without producing a deformed breast (Clough et al. 1990).

Once remodelled, the breast is smaller and higher with a narrower base, but its form remains normal. A symmetrising procedure is frequently required on the contralateral breast. This may, if practical, be performed at the same operative sitting, but is usually performed some months after completion of all treatments, particularly radiotherapy.

The techniques used early in our experience included superior-pedicle, inverted-T mammaplasty, from plastic surgery, followed by J- and L-mammaplasties.

Other techniques have been developed over time and are adapted to specific tumour locations, including: inferior pedicle (for those at the junction of the superior quadrants), lateral mammaplasty (for laterally-based tumours), and the omega and V techniques (for superior and superomedial cancers, respectively). Medial tumours can be addressed with the mirror image of lateral mammaplasty: medial mammaplasty. Finally, techniques specifically intended for tumours around the IMF have been developed in order to minimise scarring and, if possible, symmetrisation on the contralateral side.

Oncoplastic techniques may be equally performed following neoadjuvant chemotherapy. Regression of the lesion, demonstrating response of the tumour to treatment, permits breast-conserving surgery so long as one allows sufficient time to ensure that surgery can be performed without undue haemorrhagic and infectious complications. On the other hand, we found that oncoplastic procedures after primary radiotherapy made for difficult subsequent surgery and generally poorer aesthetic results. Radiotherapy is thus reserved for postoperative treatment.

It is essential to clearly mark the excision margins with clips and document the procedure to enable the radiotherapist to calculate the optimal field of irradiation

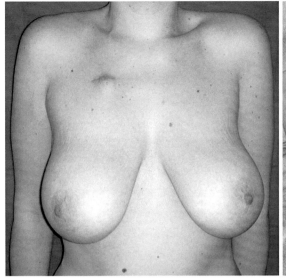

a retroareolar central tumour

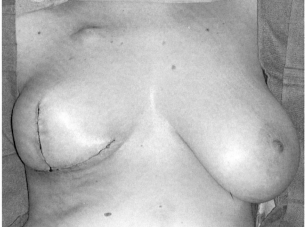

b inverted-T operative markings after neoadjuvant chemotherapy

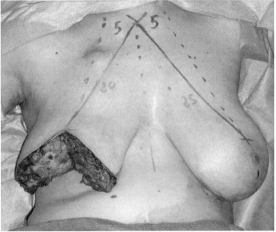

c very wide excision (weight of excised specimen: 330 g)

d reapproximation of glandular pillars and skin closure

Plate 2.2a–d   Surgical treatment of central tumours; NAC excision associated with inverted-T mammaplasty

and, if necessary the boost required, for limitation of unnecessary irradiation.

At the Institut Curie we utilise ten plastic techniques according to tumour location (Figure 2.6). These therapeutic options may also be varied depending on the form and size of the breast, existing scars, and the requirement for cutaneous excision with some tumours. The desire to avoid symmetrising the contralateral breast also influences technique selection.

Oncoplastic Breast Surgery Techniques

Superior-Pedicle, Inverted-T Mammaplasty

This technique is used for tumours at the junction of the inferior quadrants, as well as those inferolateral, inferomedial and close to the IMF (Plate 2.5).

The NAC, is supported on a superior-pedicle flap following de-epithelialisation, is elevated

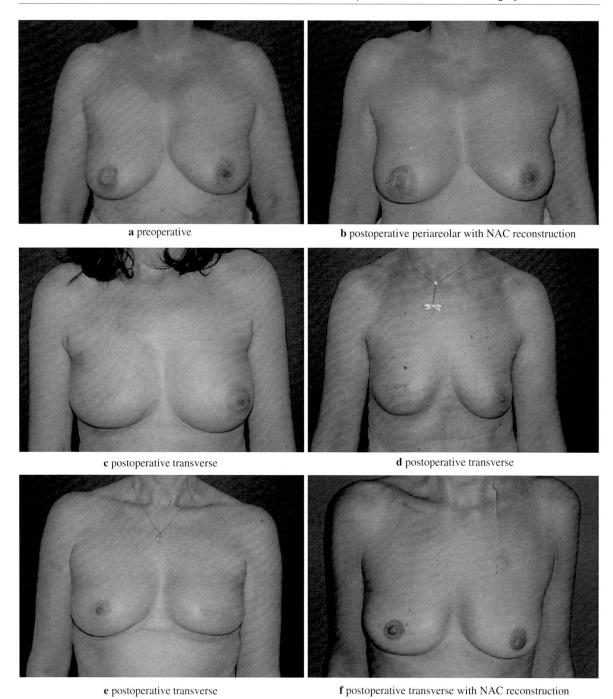

a preoperative

b postoperative periareolar with NAC reconstruction

c postoperative transverse

d postoperative transverse

e postoperative transverse

f postoperative transverse with NAC reconstruction

Plate 2.3a–f NAC excision by periareolar or transverse techniques

(Fig. 2.5b). This flap is several millimetres thick and is plicated. The mammary gland is raised from the prepectoral fascia following incision at the IMF (Fig. 2.5c). Finally, the intervening gland is excised, with a wide tumour and skin resection, at the junction of the inferior quadrants (Fig. 2.5f). The breast pillars are then reapproximated and the skin closed (Fig. 2.5g).

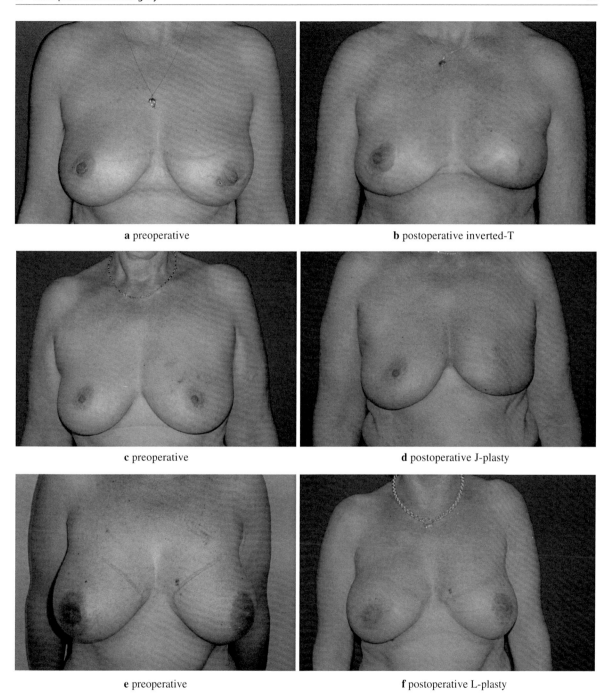

a preoperative   b postoperative inverted-T

c preoperative   d postoperative J-plasty

e preoperative   f postoperative L-plasty

Plate 2.4a–f NAC excision with plastic surgical remodelling

In this fashion, a satisfactory result can be obtained producing a smaller, higher and narrower breast (Plate 2.6).

When contralateral symmetrisation is required, it is usually done with the same technique and gland resection (with both resections being weighed), and synchronously if circumstances allow.

If the tumour is lateral or medial, a glandular rotation flap may be fashioned in order to fill the parenchymal defect (Plate 2.6).

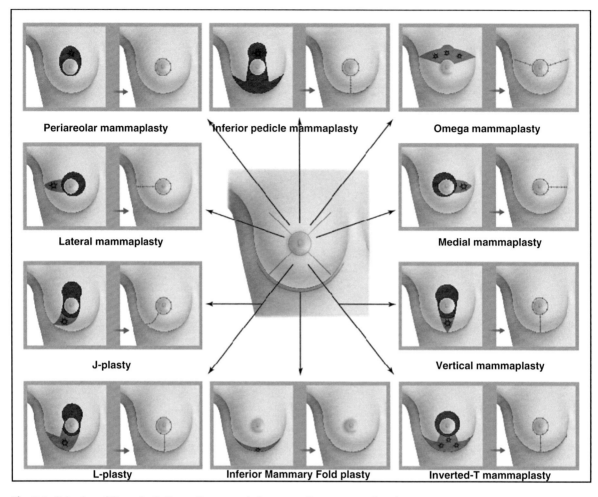

Fig. 2.6 Selection of Oncoplastic Breast Surgery technique according to tumour location

In cases of significant breast hypertrophy, an immediate NAC graft, using Thorek's technique, may be used (Thorek et al. 1989). This involves an inverted-T excision with full-thickness harvesting of the NAC, which is grafted at the summit of the vertical incision. This technique applies principally to very large and ptotic breasts where the NAC pedicle will be too long and therefore poorly vascularised (Figs. 2.7).

Vertical-Scar Mammaplasty

This technique is used for tumours at the inferior quadrant junction in smaller, non-ptotic breasts of medium size. It is the same as the inverted T, but without the IMF incision (Plate 2.8). It derives from

Lejour's vertical-scar technique (Lejour et al. 1999), and on occasion a glandular rotation flap (Plate 2.8d) is required to reconstitute the defect left after tumourectomy.

J- and L-Mammaplasty

These have similar indications to the vertical-scar and are ideal for tumours localised to the inferior or inferolateral quadrants (Plate 2.9).

The vertical incision below the areola is extended laterally, allowing limitation of the inframammary scar in large-volume breasts.

These techniques sit between a pure vertical-scar and an inverted-T mammaplasty.

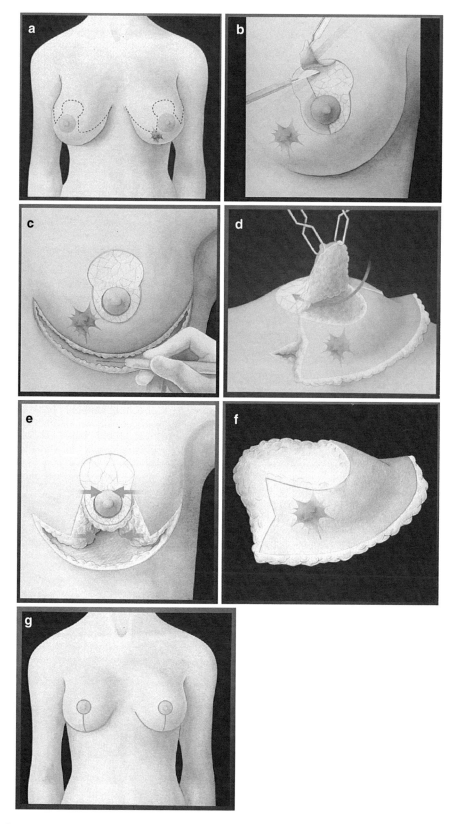

Plate 2.5a–g Schematic of inverted-T mammaplasty **a**. operative design for tumour lying within area of excision; **b**. periareolar deepithelialisation; **c**. IMF incision and dissection of the breast at the pre-pectoral plane; **d**. raising of the superiorly-based NAC flap; **e**. approximation of the breast parenchymal pillars; **f**. very wide excision specimen; **g**. resulting scars

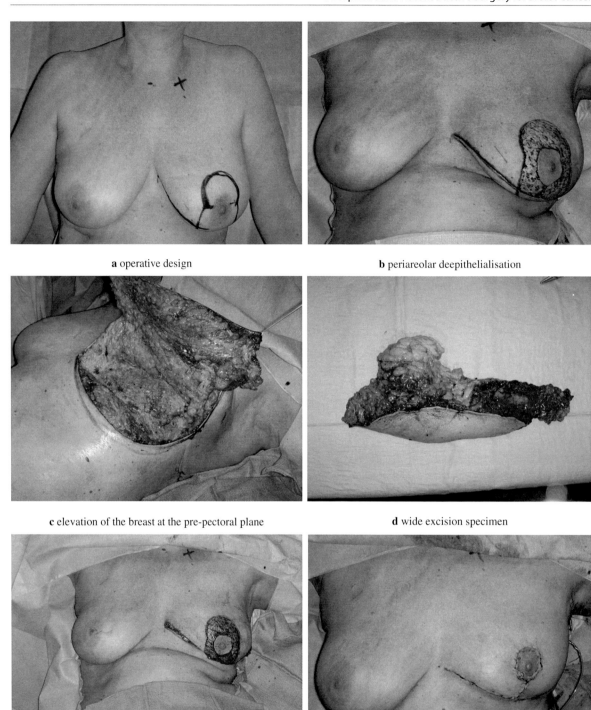

a operative design

b periareolar deepithelialisation

c elevation of the breast at the pre-pectoral plane

d wide excision specimen

e breast following tumourectomy

f on-table result

Plate 2.6a–f Inverted-T mammaplasty for inferior quadrant tumours

Inferior-Pedicle Inverted-T Mammaplasty

This technique is ideal for superior quadrant junction tumours that are close enough to the areola (particularly in ptotic breasts) (Plate 2.10). As in aesthetic surgery, it allows rejuvenation via the inferior pedicle; the zone of quadrantectomy is at the junction of the superior quadrants (Plates 2.10 and 2.11).

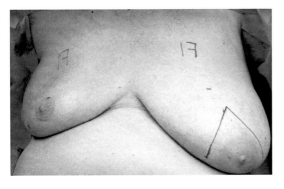

a preoperative design

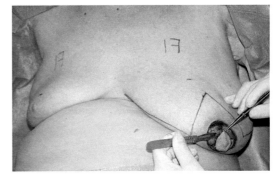

b NAC harvest as graft

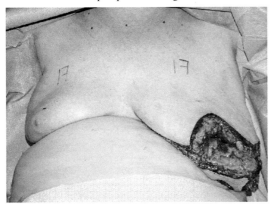

c wide tumour excision

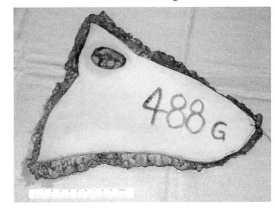

d operative specimen

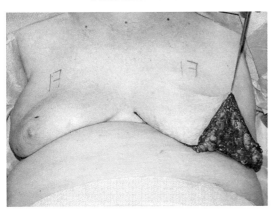

e remaining breast parenchyma

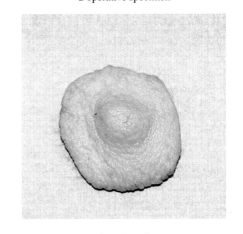

f NAC graft

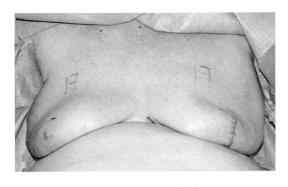

g parenchymal reconstitution

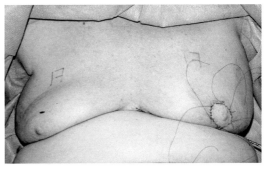

h application of the NAC graft

Plate 2.7a–h Inverted-T mammaplasty with NAC graft: Thorek technique

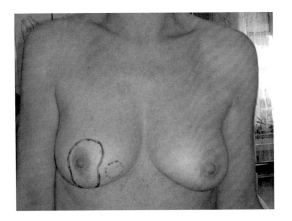

a vertical scar design for infero-medial tumour

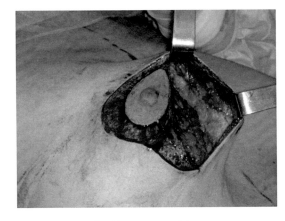

b wide tumour excision

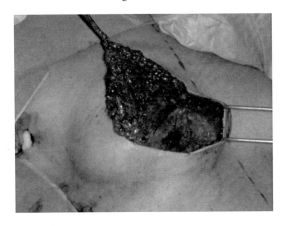

c dissection of lateral flap

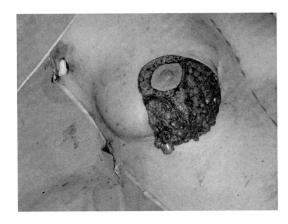

d lateral parenchymal flap

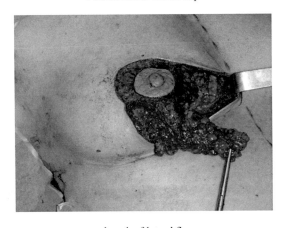

e length of lateral flap

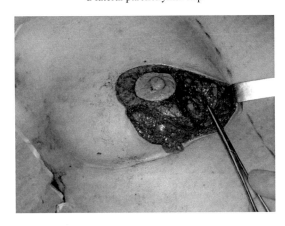

f lateral parenchymal flap advanced to fill tumourectomy defect

Plate 2.8a–f Vertical-scar technique for inferior tumours

The resulting scars are identical to those obtained with superior-pedicle inverted-T techniques (Plate 2.10f).

The resection, where tumour and skin are removed en bloc to the pectoral plane, corresponds to the future site of the NAC (Plate 2.10a). The skin is raised later-

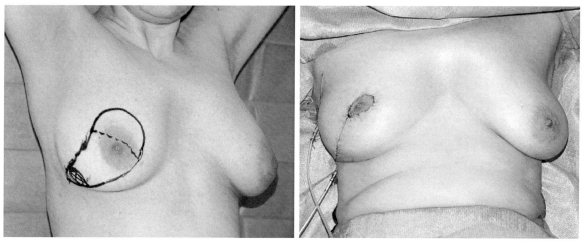

a operative design for infero-lateral tumour   **b** on-table result with NAC preservation

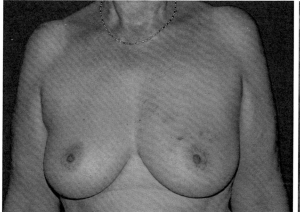
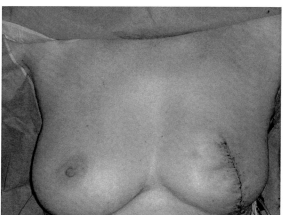

c pre-operative   **d** post-operative without NAC preservation

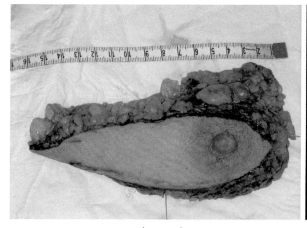
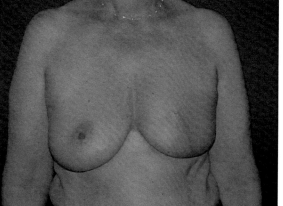

e operative specimen   **f** mature scar

Plate 2.9a–f J-mammaplasty technique

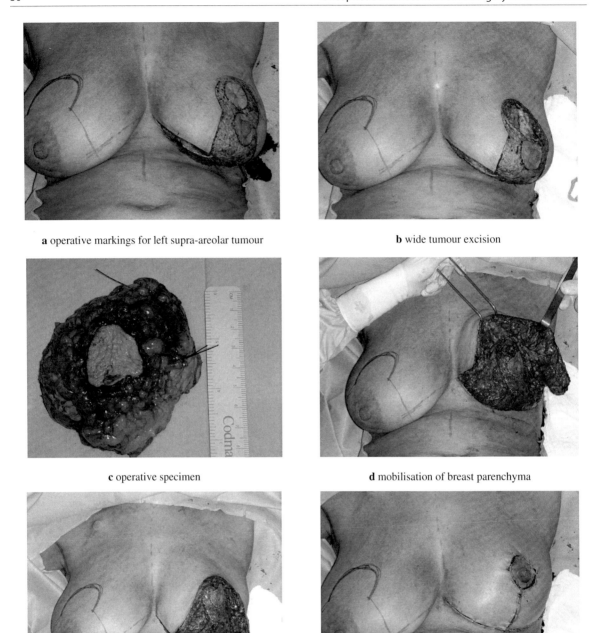

a operative markings for left supra-areolar tumour

b wide tumour excision

c operative specimen

d mobilisation of breast parenchyma

e inferiorly-pedicled NAC filling tumourectomy defect

f on-table result

Plate 2.10a–f   Inferior-pedicle mammaplasty for supra-areolar tumours

ally, leaving the NAC vascularised by an inferior pedicle (Plate 2.10d,e). Thick parenchymal flaps supplied by intercostal perforators, are then raised and transposed to fill the tumourectomy defect. Skin closure completes the procedure, and the breast is higher on the chest wall, thereby correcting ptosis (Plate 2.10f).

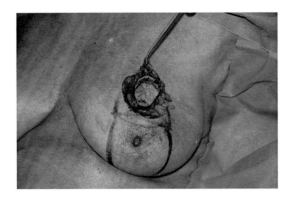

a left supra-areolar tumour incised

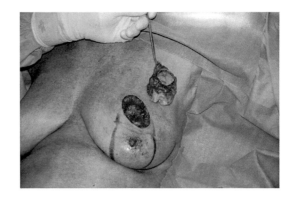

b tumour excised with overlying skin

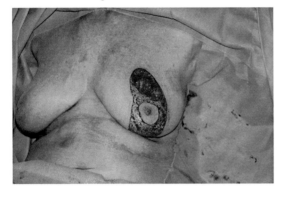

c periareolar deepithelialisation

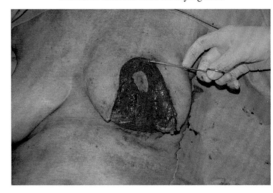

d advancement of NAC on inferior pedicle

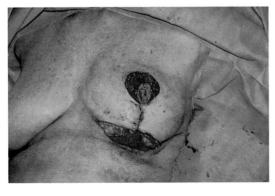

e closure of the vertical scar

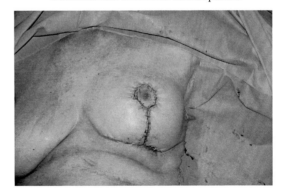

f final result

Plate 2.11a–f Inferior-pedicle mammaplasty for supra-areolar tumours

This technique facilitates the removal of any skin associated with the tumour, and gland resection is, as usual, to the prepectoral plane (Plate 2.11b).

If required, symmetrisation is more easily performed on the contralateral breast with a superior-pedicle procedure.

Periareolar Mammaplasty

This is used for tumours at the junction of the superior quadrants, as well as those superolateral or -medial, but that are close to the areola (Plates 2.12 and 2.13). The technique is comparable to the 'round block' used

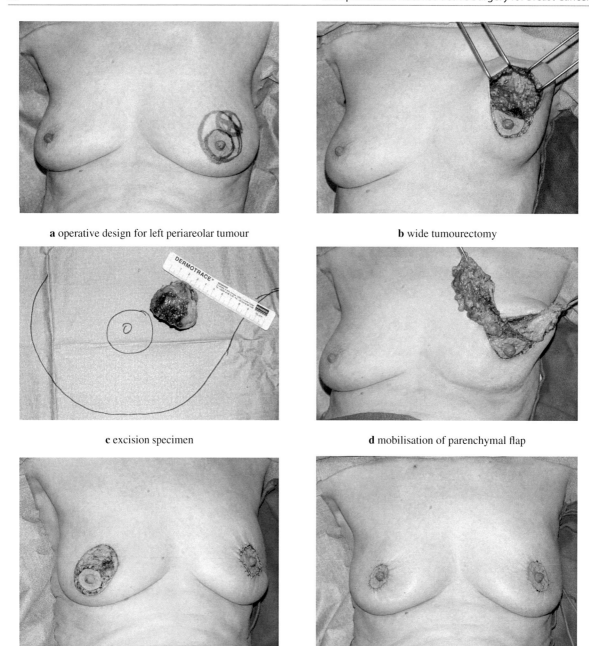

a operative design for left periareolar tumour

b wide tumourectomy

c excision specimen

d mobilisation of parenchymal flap

e closure and use of identical technique for symmetrisation

f final result

Plate 2.12a–f Periareolar technique for tumours close to the areola that require breast remodelling

in aesthetic surgery (Benelli et al. 1990). On occasion, inferior tumours close to the areola are also amenable to this technique.

Following oval periareolar de-epithelialisation, except if the tumour is adjacent to skin, the superior quadrant skin is raised and a wide tumourectomy is performed (Plate 2.12b). The glandular pillars are mobilised (Plate 2.12d), rotated and sutured to one another, allowing reconstitution of the gland, which will have a slightly narrower base. The skin is then closed, gathering the larger oval to the smaller areola to yield a pleated appearance (see Plate 2.12f).

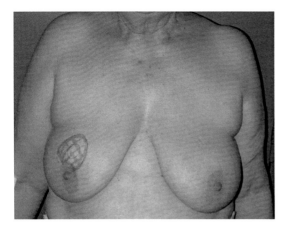

a operative design for right supra-areolar tumour

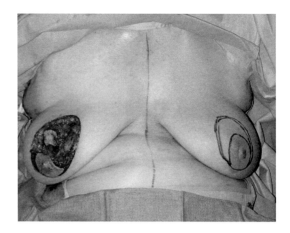

b wide tumourectomy

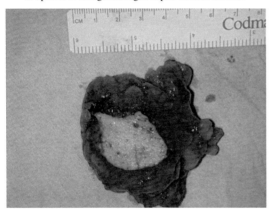

c excision specimen

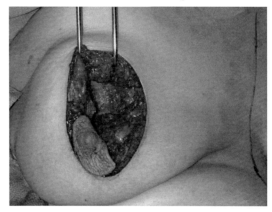

d mobilisation of breast parenchyma

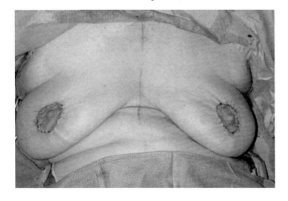

e closure and symmetrisation

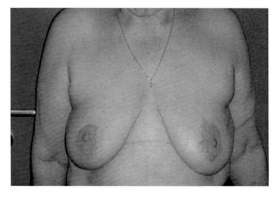

f mature result

Plate 2.13a–f Periareolar technique

Lateral Mammaplasty

Tumours at the lateral quadrant junction or, superolateral, are by far the most frequent, and this technique is therefore finding increasing use at our institution (Plates 2.14 and 2.15).

Being a simple and reliable intervention with minimal skin-gland dissection, closure is both easy and reliable.

After periareolar de-epithelialisation a cutaneoglandular incision is made to the prepectoral fascia (Plate 2.14c). This quadrantectomy removes the tumour in a wide resection (Plate 2.14d).

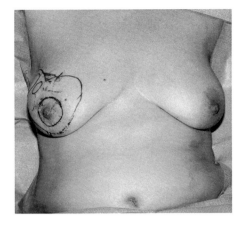

a operative design for right multifocal tumour

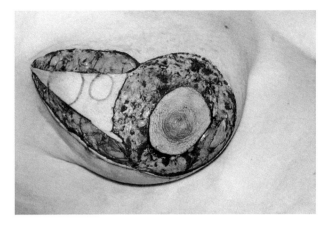

b periareolar deepithelialisation

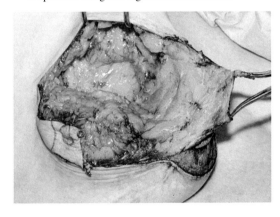

c en bloc skin and gland excision to pre-pectoral fascia

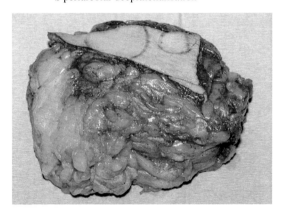

d operative specimen

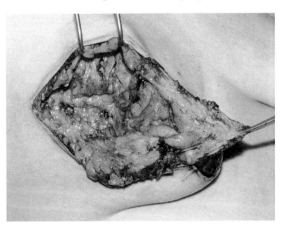

e tumourectomy defect

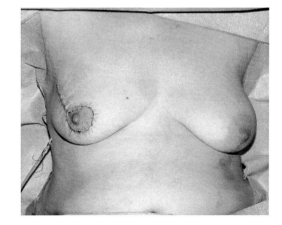

f on-table result

Plate 2.14a–f Lateral mammaplasty for tumours of the lateral quadrants

The breast is then raised, if required, at the subglandular plane, and the gland and skin are reapproximated to produce a higher breast with a narrower base.

The resulting scar is periareolar with a lateral radial extension (Plate 2.14f).

The NAC is transposed higher and more medially to avoid the inevitable inferolateral retraction following radiotherapy. Symmetrisation may be performed at the same time or later using the same technique.

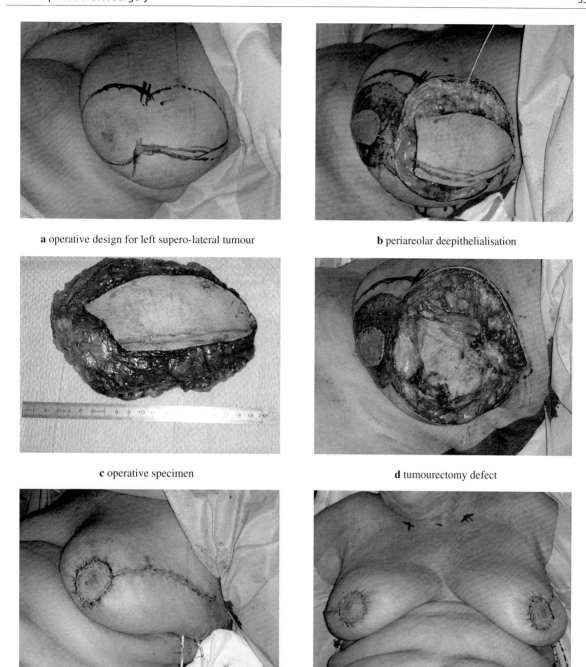

a operative design for left supero-lateral tumour

b periareolar deepithelialisation

c operative specimen

d tumourectomy defect

e wound closure

f on-table result with symmetrisation

Plate 2.15a–f Lateral mammaplasty for tumourectomy and immediate symmetrisation

One can sometimes stagger the skin and gland incisions to prevent the cutaneous scar from riding too high. A glandular flap is used to fill the deficit produced by the tumourectomy.

Omega Mammaplasty

This technique is ideal for superior quadrant and superomedial tumours, particularly in ptotic breasts

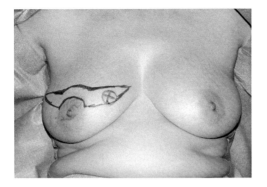

a operative design for right supero-medial tumour

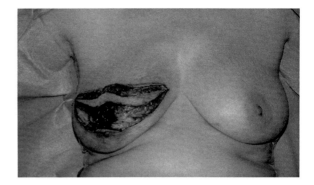

b incision

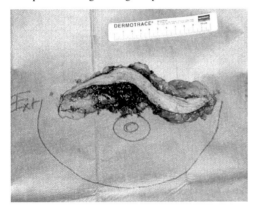

c operative specimen

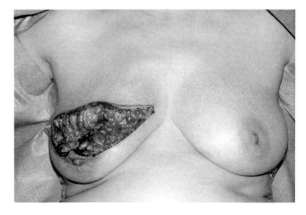

d tumourectomy defect

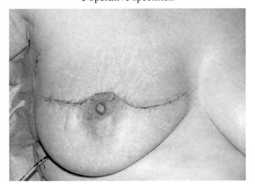

e wound closure

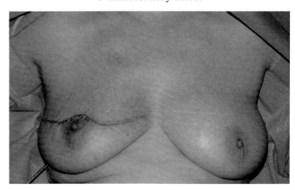

f on-table result showing good form and volume

Plate 2.16a–f Omega mammaplasty

(Plate 2.16a) that involves an en bloc excision of skin, gland and tumour, which is widely resected to the prepectoral plane (Plate 2.16).

The inferior quadrants and NAC are elevated and attached to the upper part following excision.

This simple technique allows the management, without extensive skin-gland dissection, of tumours in diffi-cult locations (superomedial, particularly those situated very high) in combination with ptosis correction.

The skin associated with the tumour is removed and the resulting scar invariably improved by radiotherapy.

Contralateral breast symmetrisation is generally performed with an alternative technique (Plate 2.17).

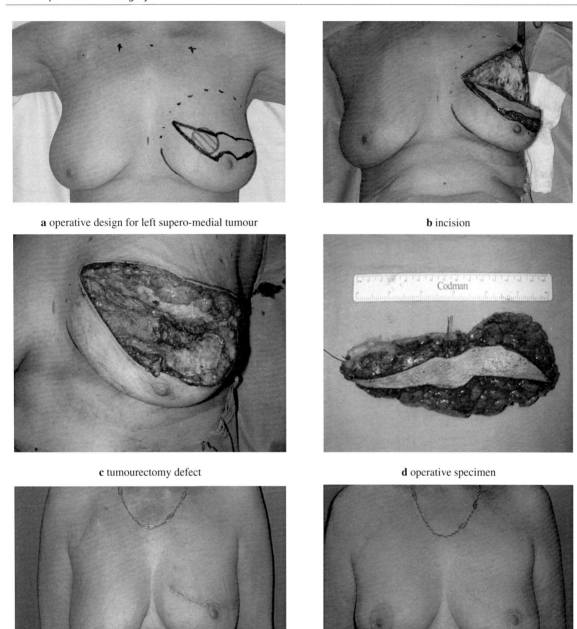

a operative design for left supero-medial tumour

b incision

c tumourectomy defect

d operative specimen

e early result

f result after radiotherapy with vertical scar contra-lateral symmetrisation

Plate 2.17a–f   Omega technique and vertical-scar contra-lateral symmetrisation

Medial Mammaplasty (Plate 18)

The medial mammaplasty technique for medial tumours is conceptually equivalent to the lateral mammaplasty. It is, however, more challenging due to the much reduced tissue volume and relative immobility of the inferomedial breast. Furthermore, inferomedial tumours frequently require skin to be included with the tumour resection.

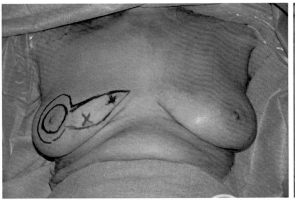

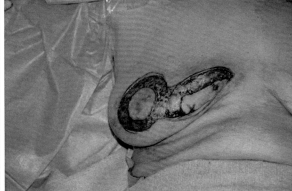

a operative design for right bifocal medial pole cancer

b peri-areolar deepithelialisation and incision

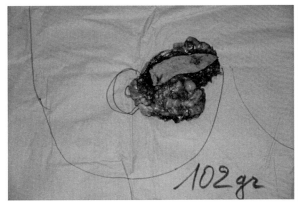

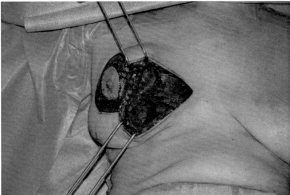

c excision specimen

d tumourectomy defect

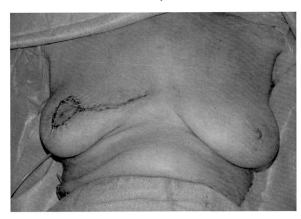

e on-table result

Plate 2.18a–e medial mammaplasty technique with NAC repositioning and direct closure

Periareolar de-epithelialisation and radial extension for tumour excision are similarly performed. Because of the relative paucity of gland, however, suture of the adjacent breast pillars is not always possible. In these cases, a lateral cutaneoglandular flap (Plate 2.19) is raised by incising the inframammary fold and then rotated medially into the defect. As usual, the resulting breast has a narrower base and sits higher on the thoracic wall.

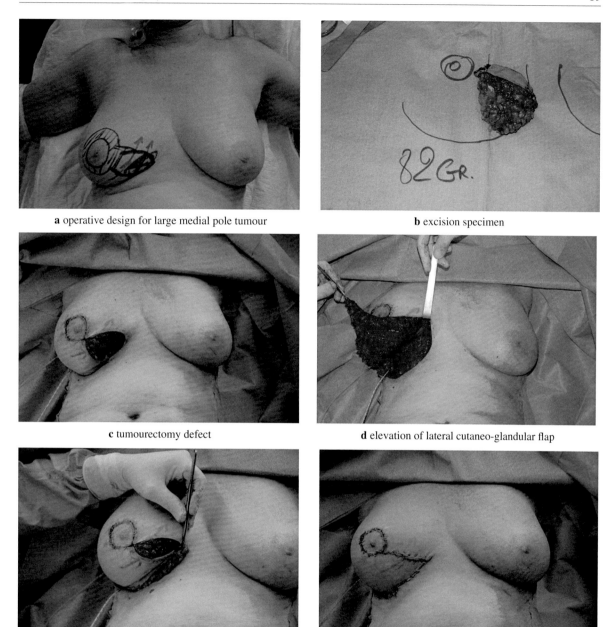

a operative design for large medial pole tumour

b excision specimen

c tumourectomy defect

d elevation of lateral cutaneo-glandular flap

e rotation of flap

f on-table result

Plate 2.19a–f medial mammaplasty technique with lateral cutaneo-glandular rotation flap

Inferior Mammary Fold (IMF) Mammaplasty

Designed for tumours at or slightly above the IMF, this technique makes it possible to avoid significant scars (as with the inverted-T) by lowering the IMF. This simple technique can be associated when required with one or two adipodermal flaps (derived from Holström's technique, Chapter 4) if the glandular deficit is significant (Plate 2.20).

When the tumour occupies the IMF it is completely excised, taking a good centimetre above and below the fold for adequate margins.

Excision is performed en bloc to the prepectoral fascia, and the two wound edges are attached to each other; this reduces segment 3, so it cannot be used with short areola–IMF distances, but it is useful for modifying the lower breast pole, particularly when ptotic.

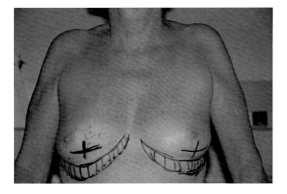

a operative design for bilateral lower pole tumours

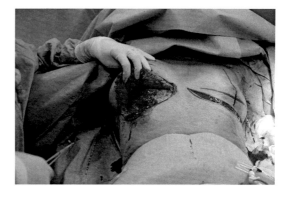

b excision of right infero-medial tumour

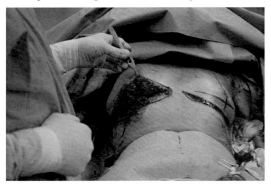

c use of lateral parenchymal flap to preserve volume

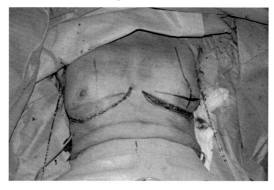

d right tumourectomy

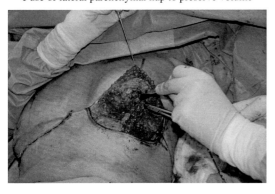

e right medial parenchymal flap rotated to preserve projection

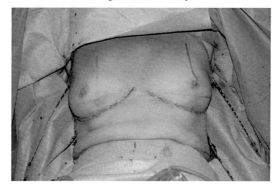

f on-table result

Plate 2.20a–f IMF mammaplasty for tumours close to the inframammary fold

Review of Oncoplastic Breast Surgery

We reviewed 299 consecutive breast cancer patients treated between 1985 and 2003 at the Institut Curie. This series concerned patients with high tumour-to-breast volume ratios or tumours in difficult locations. Mammaplasty allowed sufficient oncological resection and the avoidance of poor aesthetic results.

The mean age was 52 years (29–91)

The tumour was within the superior quadrants in 17%, medial in 19%, lateral in 20%, and at the inferior quadrant junction in 43%. The mean weight of resection in our recent series was 232 g (range 10–1,700) (Staub 2008). Symmetrisation was performed immediately in 64% and at a later date in the remainder (approximately six months after irradiation).

The mean size of these lesions was 30 mm (range 4–80) before any treatment and 25 mm (0–80 mm) after neoadjuvant chemotherapy.

The tumours were T_0 ($n = 18\%$), T_1 ($n = 18\%$), T_2 ($n = 54\%$) and larger in 10%. Skin involvement was seen in four patients.

Histopathological types included carcinoma in situ ($n = 25\%$); infiltrating ductal with or without with an intraductal component ($n = 63\%$); infiltrating lobular ($n = 6\%$); and a single case of Paget's disease.

Mammaplasty was necessary in 50% to avoid mastectomy, because of tumour location or breast deformation. In 15% it was dictated by sheer tumour volume, and in the remainder it was due to a combination of location and anticipated deformity.

Discussion

Involved excision margins are one of the principal factors in local tumour recurrence. Some authors, including Veronesi, have therefore suggested that extra-wide "quadrantectomies" should always be performed; however, the deformities they can produce are difficult to accept at an aesthetic level.

Mammaplasties for cancer have therefore allowed reconciliation of the dual objectives of clear excision margins and aesthetically acceptable remodelling of the breast.

In our series, despite wide glandular resections with a mean weight of > 200 g, the rate of good or very good results has been very high (> 85%).

These interventions are certainly most easily adapted to medium- or large-volume breasts, but may on occasion be used effectively in smaller breasts too. The rate of breast deformity would therefore be much increased in the absence of the various techniques described above.

The scar burden, sometimes significant, is often well accepted when the alternative is a radical mastectomy, and radiotherapy usually improves the long-term appearance with little fibrous reaction. It is paradoxical that patients will often complain more about the symmetrised than the treated side, as irradiation minimises hypertrophic scarring.

The advantages of such "Oncoplastic Breast Surgery" are clear:

– Quality of excision margins

– Increase in breast-conserving treatments
– Reduction in adverse aesthetic sequelae following conservation
– Overall survival and five-year recurrence rates that are identical to standard conservative surgery
– Immediate symmetry without other reconstructive gestures

On the other hand, the duration of intervention is lengthened, and specifically trained surgeons are required to obtain optimal results.

Conclusion

The integration of oncoplastic techniques into breast cancer surgery has allowed us to reduce the rate of mastectomy and the adverse sequelae of breast-conserving surgery.

Mastectomies are avoided in instances of sizeable tumour volume, difficult tumour location, or high tumour-to-breast volume ratios.

These limits may also be extended by diminishing the preoperative tumour volume using a medical treatment (chemotherapy or hormonal therapy). It is important, however, to understand that radiotherapy must only be used postoperatively, because it greatly increases poor aesthetic results when used preoperatively.

References

Benelli L (1990) A new periareolar mammoplasty: the "round block" technique. Aesth Plast Surg 14:93–100

Clough KB, Soussaline M, Campana F, et al. (1990) Plastie mammaire associée à une irradiation: traitement conservateur des cancers du sein localisés dans les quadrants inférieurs. Ann Chir Plast Esth 35:117–22

Fisher B, Anderson S, Redmond CK, et al. (1995) Reanalysis and results after 12 years of follow-up in a randomized clinical trial comparing total mastectomy with or without irradiation in the treatment of breast cancer. N Engl J Med 333:1456–61

Fisher B, Dignam J, Wolmark N, et al. (1998) Lumpectomy and radiation therapy for the treatment of intraductal breast cancer: findings from National Surgical Adjuvant Breast and Bowel Project B-17. J Clin Oncol 16:441–52

Jacobson JA, Danforth DN, Cowan KH, et al. (1995) Ten-year results of a comparison of conservation with mastectomy in the treatment of stage I and II breast cancer. N Engl J Med 332:907–11

Lejour M (1999) Vertical mammoplasty update and appraisal of late results. Plast Recons Surg 104:764–81

Solin LJ, Kurtz J, Fourquet A, et al. (1996) Fifteen-year results of breast conserving treatment and definitive breast irradiation for the treatment of ductal carcinoma in situ of the breast. J Clin Oncol 14:754–63

Staub G, Fitoussi A, Falcou M-C, Salmon RJ (2008) Breast cancer surgery: use of mammaplasty. Results from Institute Curie. Ann Chir Plast Aesthet 53:124–34

Thorek M (1989) Possibilities in the reconstruction of the human form. Aesth Plast Surg 13:55–8

van Dongen JA, Voogd AC, Fentiman IS, et al. (2000) Long term results of a randomized trial comparing breast-conserving therapy with mastectomy. European Organization for Research and Treatment of Cancer 10801 trial. J Natl Cancer Inst 92:1143–50

Prostheses and Expanders

Introduction

Breast augmentation with prosthetic implants is a procedure that dates back to the 1950s. Silicone quickly became the preferred implant material because of its inert properties and good tolerance. Techniques and the prostheses themselves have evolved significantly over the years:

– Initial techniques made use of the injection of silicone liquid directly into the tissues, but serious complications ensued including cysts, ulceration and deformation.
– The first subcutaneous implants (Edgerton and McClary 1958) induced severe fibrosis, as they were made of a permeable material.
– Double-lumen implants then became popular. These comprised an internal membrane containing silicone with a smooth outer membrane: the intervening space being filled with saline. They were abandoned at the beginning of the 1990s due to technical problems, particularly leakage.
– Implants with silicone as both shell and filler appeared in 1963 (Cronin 1963) in the form of an anatomically shaped prosthesis with a Dacron patch attached to the posterior surface. Numerous modifications of this design have since appeared.

Saline-filled silicone-shelled prostheses became commercially available around the same time (Arion 1965), and there are different types:
– Implants prefilled by the manufacturers
– Implants filled during the operation with a volume recommended by the manufacturers

– Implants that allow progressive expansion after surgical insertion; this expansion being performed regularly over several weeks or months until the optimal volume is reached (this type being known as expanders)

Health concerns

The first questions about the harmlessness of silicone-filled prostheses surfaced in the United States at the end of the 1970s, following descriptions of periprosthetic leakage (Baker et al. 1982). Cases of unexpected autoimmune diseases, such as scleroderma, in patients with these prostheses were reported (van Nunen et al. 1982; Sergott et al. 1986), in addition to suggestions of potential carcinogenesis, which limited the marketing of these implants to breast reconstruction only with their use being prohibited for aesthetic surgery from 1992.

In France, the authorities banned silicone prostheses whilst awaiting confirmation of their safety. Other European countries, however, rapidly reintroduced them. In France, it took until November 2000, when a *New England Journal of Medicine* meta-analysis confirmed the absence of any link between silicone implants and either autoimmune diseases or cancer (Janowsky et al. 2000), before the restrictions on their use were lifted. The FDA in America took even longer, only lifting the moratorium in December 2006.

Types of Prostheses

As both the form and volume of the breast are highly variable, so there are numerous shapes and sizes of

A. Fitoussi et al., *Oncoplastic and Reconstructive Surgery for Breast Cancer,*
DOI: 10.1007/978-3-642-00144-4_3, © Springer-Verlag Berlin Heidelberg 2009

prostheses. The aim of implant-based reconstruction is to match the contralateral breast as closely as possible.

Today's prostheses are all silicone-shelled. Two types of silicone are used, with different polymerisation temperatures giving different physical properties: one for the shell and one for the filler.

For the shell, silicone liquid is applied to a mould by immersion. This operation is repeated several times, resulting in a multilaminated shell (most manufacturers use between three and seven layers) that is thicker and thus more resistant than older versions.

The addition of a layer of silicone with a different composition (known as the barrier coat) among these layers reduces transudation of the internal contents (known as "gel bleed") across the shell.

With respect to the filler, saline or silicone gel can be used; the latter being available in a range of viscosities, known as cohesivity, allowing implants of differing flexibility and feel.

Expanders are implants with silicone shells that are filled to different volumes with saline.

Prostheses can be differentiated according to their shape, texture and content.

Shape

Round Prostheses

These are hemispherical with a flat base and the volume is determined by two dimensions: diameter and projection. For a similar volume, a high-profile, i.e., more projecting, prosthesis has a narrower base than a low-profile and vice versa.

Anatomical Prostheses

These are shaped like the breast itself, being wider at the bottom and are characterised by volume, width, height and projection. The height/projection ratio allows high and low prostheses to be differentiated.

Asymmetric Prostheses

These are a further development of anatomical prostheses that have concave posterior surfaces, allowing

them to mould to the thoracic wall. They are much wider than they are tall, have more inferolateral projection, and better fill the medial part of the reconstructed breast. There are only two heights, tall and short and they are unique to each side (Fitoussi 2005).

Texture

Modifications to the envelope appeared at the end of the 1980s in an attempt to reduce the phenomena of migration and capsular contracture. The manufacturers produced different textures, but improvements resulting from these different textures remain moderate.

During the course of implant manufacture, texturisation is performed prior to filling, when the shell is completed. There are different shell coats:

– Smooth: these have the greatest risk of migration, rotation and capsular contracture
– Microtextured: by foam imprints (Mentor) or salt crystallisation (Inamed)
– Macrotextured: also known as highly textured, produced by silicone saturation after salination (McGhan)

Content

Early prostheses were filled with liquid silicone, which gave them a consistency similar to that of a normal breast, but because of problems with leaks, manufacturers developed silicone gels that differed in viscocity or cohesiveness.

These "cohesive" gels are characterised by low migratory ability through a standardised funnel, additionally resulting in improved retention of the implant.

One major inconvenience of this is the fixed appearance and feel that some prostheses may have. There are therefore gels with differing cohesivenesses, for different situations and patient choice.

Degree of fill is an important parameter because it allows a further parameter of refinement. Underfilling improves the feel, but increases the sensation of "waves", the appearance of visible ripples, and shortens the life of the implant due to fold flaws. Overfilling reduces the suppleness of the implant and tends to be reserved for expanders.

Indications

Indications for immediate breast reconstruction by prosthesis include:

– Prophylactic mastectomies in cases of proven genetic mutation or a family history suggesting such a mutation
– Extensive ductal carcinoma in situ where radiotherapy is not planned postoperatively
– Some mastectomies for recurrence after conservative treatment where the tissues allow
– Small infiltrating carcinomata with a morphology favourable to prosthesis use and for which adjuvant radiotherapy is not envisaged

Immediate reconstruction is not advised if postoperative radiotherapy is planned or likely, except in particular cases discussed under the aegis of the MDT.

Contralateral symmetrisation, when necessary, is performed either simultaneously or at a second stage, depending upon the patient's individual circumstances.

Surgical Techniques

Whether reconstruction is immediate or delayed, the operative designs are first made with the patient awake and standing. The patient is installed on an articulated table that allows a semi-seated position during the procedure.

In both cases the implants are placed submuscularly.

Immediate Breast Reconstruction (IBR)

A complete musculofascial pocket is created by lateral and inferolateral dissection of the pectoralis minor and serratus anterior muscles (Plates 3.1–3.2).

If indicated, mastectomy is performed with conservation of the skin envelope, but the NAC is included in the resection with a fusiform incision that is more oblique inferiorly (Fig. 3.1a, b, c, d and e).

Dissection of the implant pocket commences at the lateral border of the pectoralis major. Submuscular dissection is facilitated by a lighted retractor and continues to the medial insertions, which may require some division. Dissection should not pass too high on the thorax in order to prevent the risk of a high-riding prosthesis (Fig. 3.1f).

The lateral part of the pocket comprises pectoralis minor and serratus anterior. Pectoralis minor is raised from the thoracic wall commencing at its medial border, continues in contact with a rib, and proceeds laterally. The intercostal muscles are adjacent and inadvertent dissection beneath the latter, which are in contact with the parietal pleura, risks a pneumothorax. The inferolateral pocket is formed by the serratus anterior muscle and inferiorly by the fascia anterior to the rectus abdominis (Clough et al. 2005) or the conjoint fascia of the rectus-external oblique muscles (Fig. 3.2a–c).

With the patient in a seated position, dissection proceeds inferiorly between the rectus sheath and the superficial fascia. An adipocutaneous abdominal advancement flap (AAF) is thus created, which contributes to ptosis of the reconstructed breast (Fig. 3.2d,e).

The IMF is preserved during mastectomy, but dissection of the implant pocket leads to separation of its deep attachment. It is therefore imperative to fix the neo-IMF, in part to limit the inferior pocket and in part to assure the shape of the reconstruction (Plate 3.2 e and f).

Trial prostheses are used prior to the definitive implant. Once the definitive prosthesis is in place, the muscular pocket is closed over a suction drain by suturing the lateral border of pectoralis major to the medial border of pectoralis minor (Plate 3.3a–c).

A second suction drain is placed in the mastectomy pocket (Plate 3.3d–f).

Delayed Breast Reconstruction (DBR)

This is undertaken several months after completion of any adjuvant treatment. It is conveniently associated with a contralateral symmetrising procedure, which may be either reduction or prosthetic augmentation.

The mastectomy scar is excised and always sent for histopathological evaluation.

The retropectoral plane is most often limited by its external border. It is followed medially and superolaterally. Inferiorly, the implant is subcutaneous, and an abdominal advancement flap is routinely raised with fixation of the neo-IMF (Plates 3.4 and 3.5).

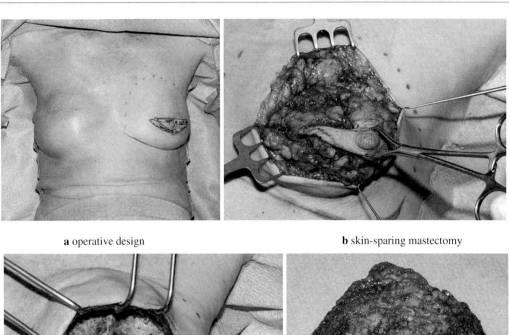

a operative design   b skin-sparing mastectomy

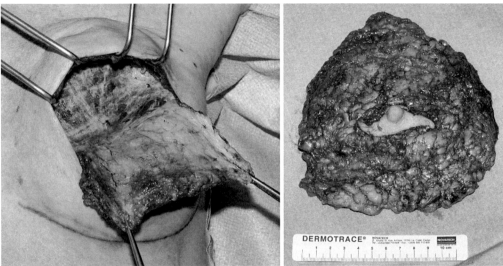

c conservation of the pectoral fascia   d mastectomy specimen

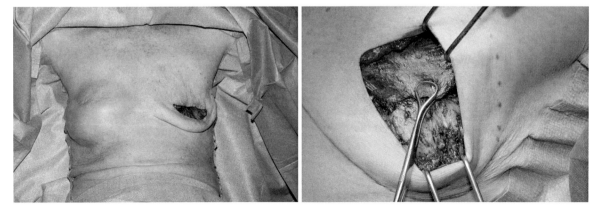

e. preservation of the skin envelope   f dissection of the lateral border of pectoralis major

Plate 3.1a–f Implant-based IBR; mastectomy with skin envelope preservation

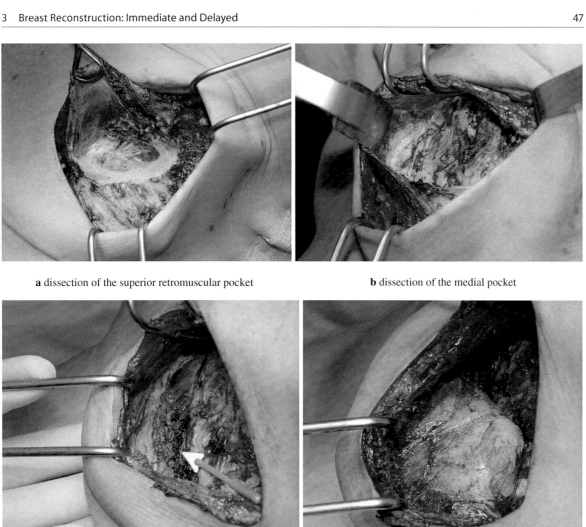

a dissection of the superior retromuscular pocket   **b** dissection of the medial pocket

c incision of the superficial thoracoabdominal fascia   **d** inner surface of the AAF flap

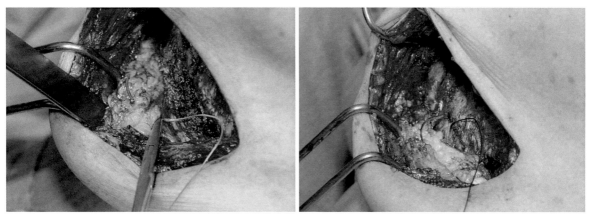

e suture insertion into the fascia   **f** elavation and suture of the flap to the periosteum

Plate 3.2a–f   Dissection of the retromuscular pocket and abdominal advancement flap (AAF)

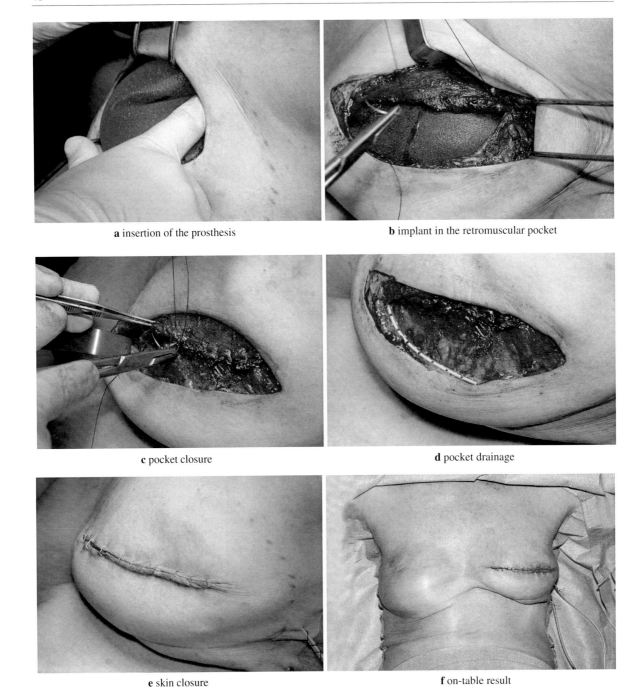

a insertion of the prosthesis

b implant in the retromuscular pocket

c pocket closure

d pocket drainage

e skin closure

f on-table result

Plate 3.3a–f IBR by prosthesis; placement of the retromuscular prosthesis and closure

Abdominal Advancement Flap and the IMF

Following mastectomy, retromuscular dissection continues inferiorly, superficial the rectus sheath to allow tailoring of an adipocutaneous flap that is advanced from the abdominal wall (Plate 3.6).

Incision of the superficial fascia, from within, across the entire width of the dissection improves the laxity of these tissues, allowing the creation of a neo-IMF when the abdominal advancement flap is lifted and then fixed with interrupted, braided, absorbable sutures to the costal periosteum below the level of the contralateral IMF.

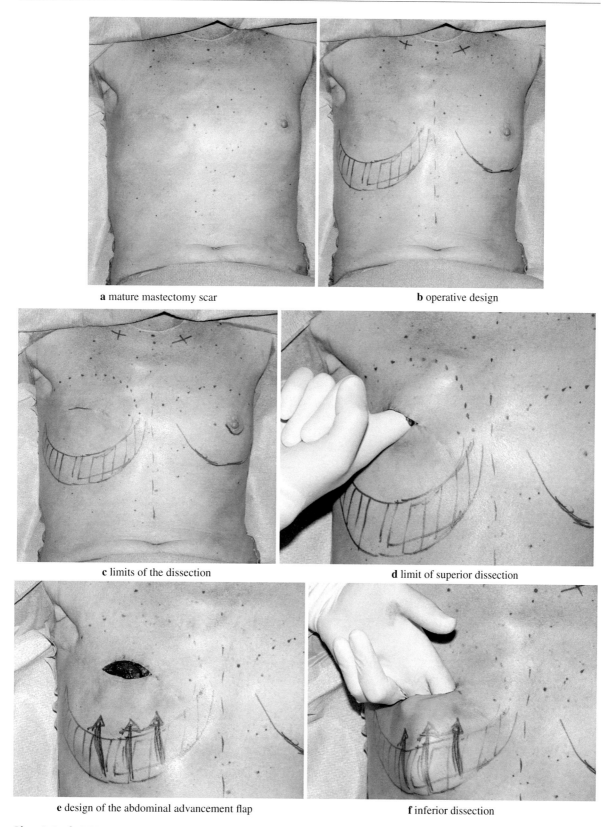

a mature mastectomy scar

b operative design

c limits of the dissection

d limit of superior dissection

e design of the abdominal advancement flap

f inferior dissection

Plate 3.4a–f DBR by prosthesis; creation of the retromuscular pocket and abdominal advancement flap

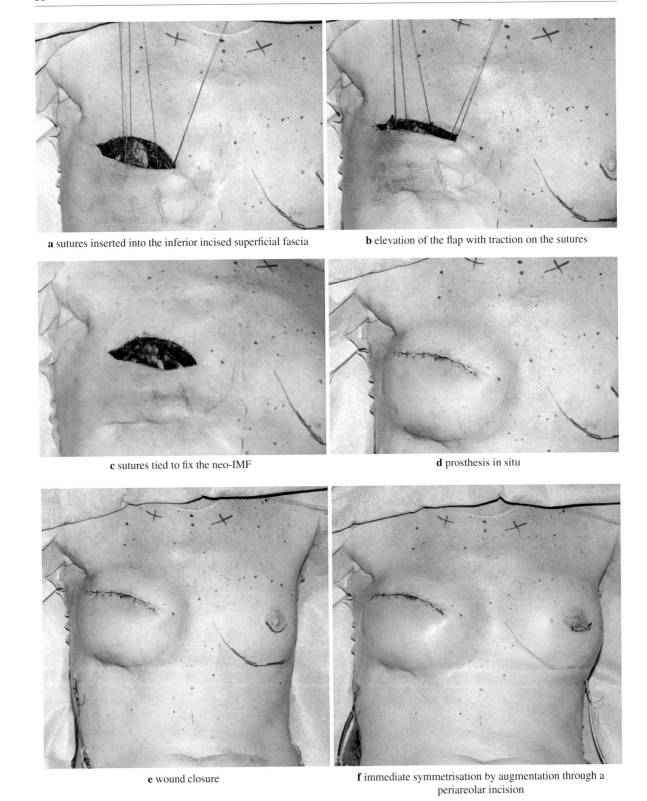

a sutures inserted into the inferior incised superficial fascia

b elevation of the flap with traction on the sutures

c sutures tied to fix the neo-IMF

d prosthesis in situ

e wound closure

f immediate symmetrisation by augmentation through a periareolar incision

Plate 3.5a–f DBR by prosthesis; creation of the neo-IMF and immediate symmetrisation

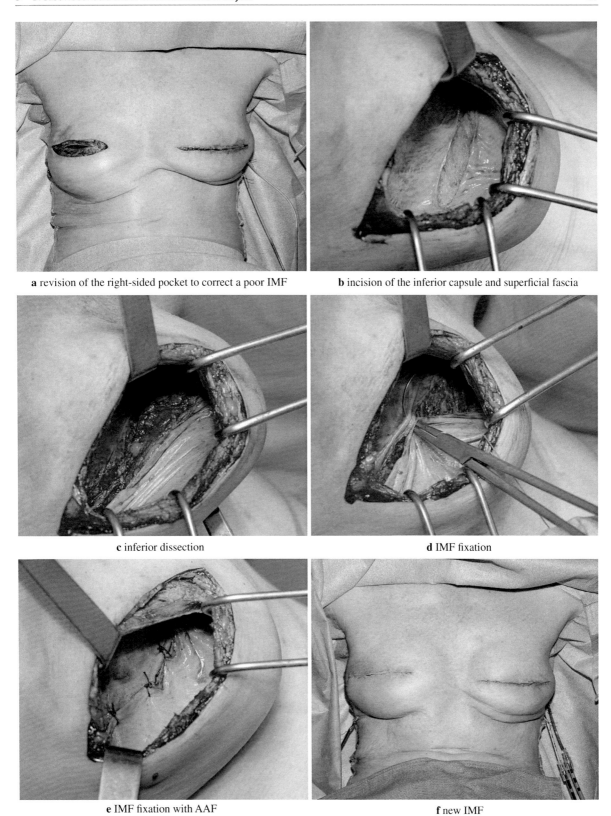

a revision of the right-sided pocket to correct a poor IMF

b incision of the inferior capsule and superficial fascia

c inferior dissection

d IMF fixation

e IMF fixation with AAF

f new IMF

Plate 3.6a–f   Use of the abdominal advancement flap for improved IMF definition

The solidity of this anchorage underpins the stability of the reconstruction (Figs. 3.6a–d). One central stitch fixes the level of the inferior fascia, then 4–6 stitches placed medially and laterally allow the formation of a curved neo-IMF. The neo-IMF is placed 1–2 cm lower than its final position because of the elevation that routinely occurs in the following months.

This technique of raising an AAF provides both a solid, new IMF and additional tissue allowing the aesthetic outcome to be improved. It also reduces the revisions required for prosthesis-based reconstruction and the need for musculocutaneous flaps.

Reconstruction of the IMF is fundamental if optimal aesthetic results are to be achieved in implant-based breast reconstruction (Figs. 3.6f). Support for this concept is wide and modifications have been suggested by other authors (Wechselberger et al. 2003; Pennisi 1977; May et al. 1987); however, histological and anatomical descriptions of the IMF remain controversial.

The existence of a suspensory inframammary ligament has been discussed (Maillard and Garey 1987; Bayati and Seckel 1995; Boutros et al. 1998), although others have described a reflection of the superficial fascia (Muntan et al. 2000) and incorrectly concluded that its superficial extension originates from the IMF (Nava et al. 1998).

In fact, it appears that the inframammary fold is a zone of adherence between the superficial fascia (incorrectly named the "deep leaf of the superficial fascia") and the subcutaneous tissues (Lockwood 1991).

Complications

Complications may be divided into those that occur "early" (in the first two postoperative months including haematomata, infections, thrombosis, pulmonary embolism etc.) or "late" thereafter, as described below by frequency of occurrence.

They are more frequent after IBR than DBR (Edgerton and McClary 1958) and the principal complications are as follows:

Early complications

- Haematomata (1–6%) (Cronin 1963)

These may occur in either the mastectomy or the implant pocket. There are two opposing views: some recommend immediate re-exploration, whilst others prefer an expec-

tant approach with close surveillance and echographic exploration. Treatment will be adapted to the site and the volume of the collection. We favour the latter strategy.

- Infections (0–4%) (Arion 1965)

These are uncommon and are often amenable to medical treatment with antibiotics. However, in exceptional cases it may be necessary to operate and remove the implant.

- Implant extrusion

Secondary to wound breakdown or infection, these require implant removal.

- Cutaneous necrosis

These generally appear rapidly—around the tenth postoperative day—and may require re-operation or healing by second intention if the implant is not exposed. More recently, we have been using an AAF, which allows the importation of fresh tissue and reduces wound closure tension.

Late Complications

- Adverse capsular contracture

Peri-implant capsules are the response of the organism to foreign bodies (Heymans 2005). Their precise aetiology is unclear, and likely to be multifactorial (Henriksen et al. 2005).

They are not to be confused with the thin, inner periprosthetic capsule, which appears a week after implantation and is not predictive for adverse capsular contracture (ACC: capsules may be thin but associated with a very tight contracture and vice versa).

A classification with four grades was originally described by Baker et al. (1982) and later modified:

- Grade I: normal breast appearance breast with imperceptible implant
- Grade II: breast firm, but without deformation
- Grade III: very firm breast with some visible deformation
- Grade IV: obviously deformed breast which may be painful

Clinically relevant ACC is considered as grades III and IV. These appear predominantly in the first two years and are more common after irradiation. They occur in 11% of patients at two years and 15% at five years (Clough et al. 2005, 2001), and are difficult to treat. Delayed ACC amounts to only 5% of cases. Treatment options include:

– Anterior capsulotomy, which however, has a risk of recurrence of approximately 50%
– Changing the prosthesis
– Capsulectomy
– Reconstruction with an autologous flap

ACC necessitating reintervention generally requires the notification of either a national monitoring body or the manufacturers.

• Periprosthetic creases and ripples

These are seen most often in those with thin subcutaneous tissues that echo any surface irregularities of the prosthesis.

They may be managed with fat transfer or replacement of the prosthesis with one of a different viscosity.

• Implant deflation

This phenomenon is most frequently observed in saline-filled prostheses.

The rate increases with time in a linear fashion (over 1.5% per year), and is approximately 3% at two years and 8.5% at five years (Clough et al. 2005, 2001).

• Intra- and extra-capsular implant rupture

If contained by the periprosthetic fibrous capsule, rupture is referred to as "intracapsular". Clinical signs are not particularly obvious, and it is usually first diagnosed through imaging, with the "tear drop" and "linguine" signs being well described.

When silicone escapes into the gland beyond the capsule it is known as an "extracapsular" leak (or a "siliconoma" when occurring as a discrete nodule). Clinical detection is more obvious, and radiological imaging shows a typical "snowstorm" on echography, or a diffuse hyperdensity on digital mammography. MRI remains the best technique for visualising intramammary silicone having as it does a sensitivity of 77%.

• Aging of the reconstruction

It is inevitable that prostheses display signs of aging (ruptures, leaks, gel bleed, capsules, etc.). It is impossible to determine the time that corresponds to a degree of aging that necessitates replacement of the prosthesis. A fixed, but false, belief is that the lifespan of an implant is approximately ten years. It has been shown that some implants must be changed much earlier

while others may last 15 years or more. It all depends on the type of implant used.

• Failure

Among the factors most likely to lead to failure of the reconstruction are:

– Smoking
– Previous or adjuvant radiotherapy
– Obesity

With the agreement of the patient, and if the morphology allows, it may be possible to insert a prosthesis and perform a secondary reconstruction with an autologous flap.

The two flaps most frequently used are the musculocutaneous latissimus dorsi and TRAM flaps, as detailed later in this chapter.

Surveillance and Results

The scale used to evaluate aesthetic outcome has five levels (Clough et al. 1995):

1: Very good
2: Good
3: Satisfactory
4: Poor
5: Very poor

The grade is assigned by those assisting in the consultation: the surgeon, the nurse, and the medical assistant (Clough et al. 1995, 2004; Nos et al. 1998).

At the Institut Curie, between 1990 and 1997, 360 IBR implants (57% prefilled, 43% expanders) were performed and followed prospectively in order to evaluate the overall long-term results of reconstruction. Outcome measures included symmetry, suppleness, the inframammary fold, the position and appearance of scars, and the overall result of the reconstruction (Clough et al. 2005).

The proportion of satisfactory results (grades 1–3) was 86% after one year, but this decreased rapidly to 54% at five and 36% at ten years.

Various factors were analysed (implant type, volume, mastectomy incision and age), but none were predictive with respect to the long-term aesthetic result. Only ACC was predictive for an alteration in the overall result.

Therefore, the type of prosthesis used appears to have little effect on the result. Alteration of the overall result may thus be primarily due to patient factors (tissue atrophy, changes in body weight).

It is important to emphasise that the reconstructed breast does not age in the same fashion as the contralateral breast. Thus asymmetry appears between the natural breast, which will have a tendency to undergo ptosis and enlargement, and the reconstructed breast, which remains spherical and may show periprosthetic wrinkles. Furthermore, the native breast differs from the reconstructed breast with respect to ptosis, accentua-ting any asymmetry.

Expanders

Principles and Types

These are inflatable prostheses with a silicone shell that are fitted with a self-sealing valve to allow inflation. They are filled with saline through a port.

Early implants were unreliable because of leaks around the filling port (Arion 1965). Since then the valve has been improved (Jenny 1971) enhancing their reliability.

There are two main types:

– Definitive (Becker-type, manufactured by Mentor), with a double lumen and a remote port that can be removed.
– Provisional (Allergan), which are produced in either round or anatomical configurations. The filling port is incorporated into the prosthesis and may be central or offset.

Temporary expanders are subsequently replaced with prefilled, permanent prostheses at a second operation, when the desired volume has been obtained.

Some believe that the aesthetic results obtained by this two-stage method are superior to those gained using prefilled implants (Slavin and Colen 1990; Maxwell and Falcone 1992; Gui et al. 2003).

Indications

Expanders may be used when tissue laxity is insufficient for the initial placement of a definitive prosthesis, when a flap is not possible, or when one wishes to produce a cutaneous excess to create ptosis.

In our current practice at the Curie, such implants are rarely used; we prefer either abdominal advance-ment a priori or recourse to musculocutaneous latissimus dorsi and rectus abdominis flaps.

Surgical Technique

The form and size are decided beforehand and the surgical techniques are similar to those described for prefilled prostheses, with the exception of a more inferior placement of the base of the expander as it tends to ride much higher.

The expander is inserted then inflated to a volume that does not produce tension on the scar.

Postoperative expansion is done regularly as an outpatient until a satisfactory pocket has been obtained.

Complications

These are the same as prefilled implants, but with added complications related to the filling system and the potential for leakage.

There is also a greater risk of subsequent ACC, infection and cutaneous necrosis.

In cases of the failure of expander-based breast reconstruction, it is possible (as with prefilled implants) that salvage with autologous flaps will be required, as described in other chapters.

Conclusion

Implant-based breast reconstruction is currently the technique most common employed by oncological surgeons.

Concealed behind its apparent simplicity, however, are numerous complications, as well as long-term results that are less satisfactory. However, these are variable as each patient is different and some will neither wish nor be able to undergo major autologous reconstruction.

The wide choice of prostheses offered by manufacturers allows us to choose the best implant for each patient. The ideal prosthesis will be tailor-made and present the same consistency as the contralateral breast. We have found that the abdominal advancement flap has led to improved results and is being used with increased frequency.

Clinical results of implant-based reconstructions are shown in Plates 3.7–3.10.

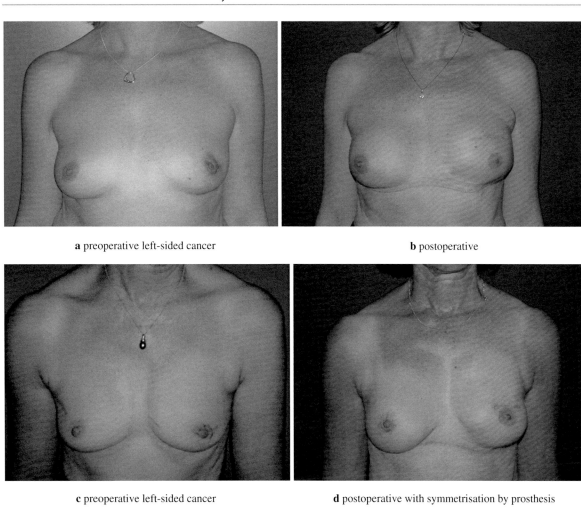

a preoperative left-sided cancer   b postoperative

c preoperative left-sided cancer   d postoperative with symmetrisation by prosthesis

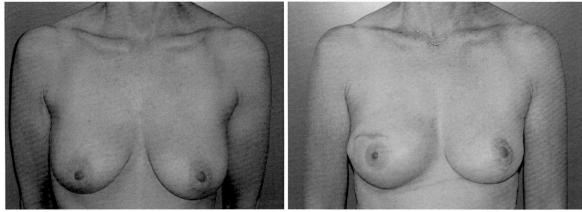

e preoperative right-sided cancer   f postoperative with vertical scar symmetrisation mastopexy

Plate 3.7a–f   Clinical results of immediate implant-based breast reconstruction

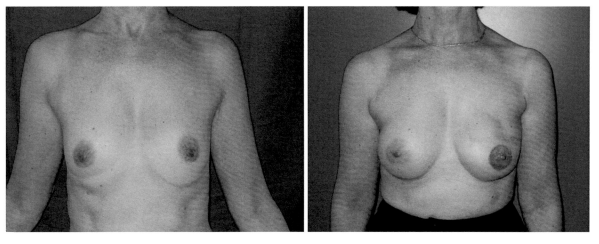

a preoperative left-sided cancer   **b** postoperative with NAC reconstruction and symmetrisation

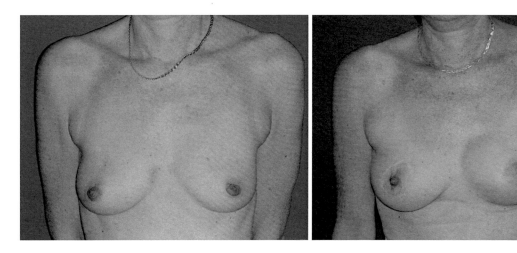

c preoperative left-sided cancer   **d** postoperative with symmetrisation

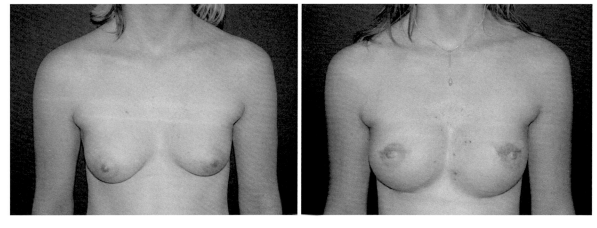

e preoperative bilateral cancer   **f** postoperative bilateral reconstruction

Plate 3.8a–f Clinical results of immediate implant-based breast reconstructions

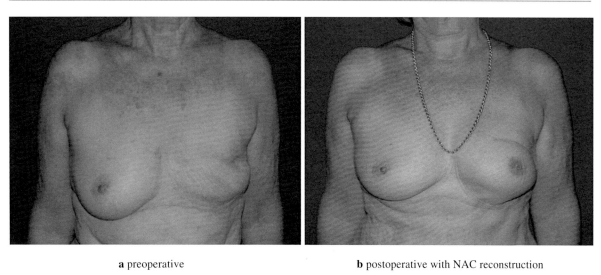

a preoperative   **b** postoperative with NAC reconstruction

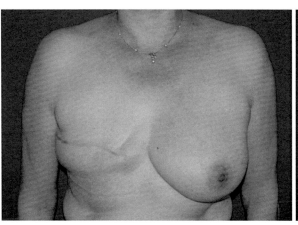
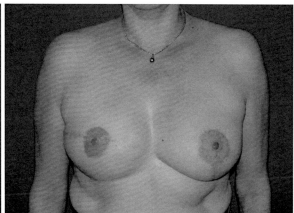

c preoperative   **d** postoperative with NAC reconstruction and inverted-T symmetrisation

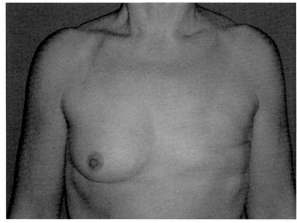
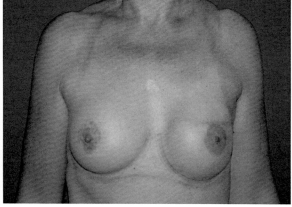

e preoperative   **f** postoperative with NAC reconstruction and symmetrisation by prosthesis

Plate 3.9a–f   Clinical results of delayed implant-based breast reconstructions

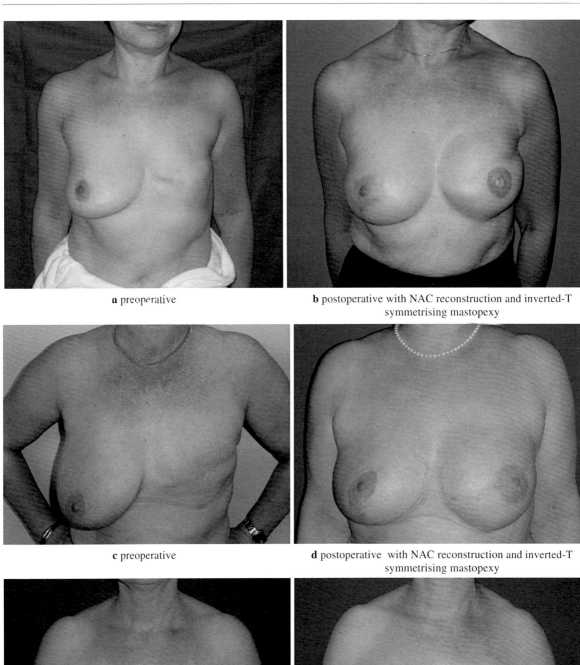

a preoperative

b postoperative with NAC reconstruction and inverted-T symmetrising mastopexy

c preoperative

d postoperative with NAC reconstruction and inverted-T symmetrising mastopexy

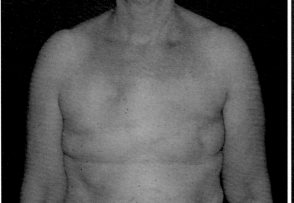

e bilateral preoperative

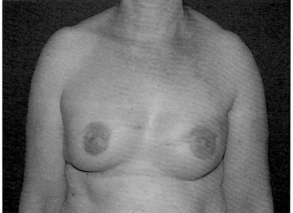

f bilateral postoperative with NAC reconstruction

Plate 3.10a–f Clinical results of delayed implant-based breast reconstruction

Latissimus Dorsi Flap

Introduction

The latissimus dorsi (LD) flap was used for the first time in 1896 by Tansini to close a mastectomy defect. However, it was the 1970s before it was used again in surgery, along with the other musculocutaneous flaps.

When the quality of the thoracic wall tissues does not allow reconstruction by prosthesis, the importation of tissue becomes essential. The latissimus dorsi flap is one of the reference techniques in such cases.

It can be used for coverage following a wide excision where direct closure is impossible, and for immediate or delayed reconstruction (either with or without a prosthesis), depending on the size of the native breast, the skin and the adipose tissue of the back.

Anatomy

The LD is one of the body's largest muscles. It originates from the lowest four ribs (and is interlinked with the serratus anterior), the lowest six thoracic and the five lumbar vertebrae, the sacrum and the posterior third of the iliac crest. This wide, fan-shaped muscle passes superolaterally past the lower scapular pole and narrows towards its insertion into the bicipital groove of the humerus.

It is a type V flap according to Mathes and Nahai's (1982) classification of muscle vascularisation, which means that it can survive solely on its principal pedicle. It is vascularised by the thoracodorsal artery, a branch of the circumflex scapular, itself a branch of the axillary artery. After entry into the muscle, the artery divides into two branches, one that descends parallel to the anterior border, the other transverse.

The venous drainage network follows the arterial pattern. The muscle is innervated by the thoracodorsal nerve, and its functions include adduction, internal rotation, and retropulsion of the arm.

Autologous Latissimus Dorsi Flap

Muscle harvest is performed with the patient in the lateral decubitus position with the arm abducted 90°, slightly rotated internally and placed on a support with a bolster beneath the axilla. It is very important to ensure correct positioning in order to avoid any points of compression and allow an unhindered dissection. The arm must not be unduly stretched in order to prevent traction on the brachial plexus. The position of the lower limbs should also be verified to avoid any compression on the lateral popliteal nerve. The surgeon must confirm this position, as he/she may be held legally responsible. Of course, contraction of the muscle should have been confirmed preoperatively (Plates 3.11 and 3.12).

First Stage: Harvest

The operative field includes the area of dorsal harvest, as well as the entire anterior thoracic area of the breast to be reconstructed (Fig. 3.11c).

We design the largest skin paddle that can be closed primarily on the back (Fig. 3.11b). This is frequently oblique anteriorly. The paddle may be designed to be horizontal if one wishes to conceal the scar in the brassiere strap.

The dorsal skin paddle is incised down to the superficial fascia (Fig. 3.11d). We have no experience of utilising iced serum or adrenaline injection at the start of the procedure in order to reduce haemorrhage.

The entire surface of the muscle is dissected following the superficial fascial plane, including the fat between fascia and muscle. The dissection is extended anteriorly, inferiorly, and beyond the superior border of the muscle to include three extensions of fat in the harvest. These fat flaps are random-pattern extensions of the latissimus dorsi (Fig. 3.11f).

There are five adipose territories in an autologous latissimus dorsi flap, which can be classified as follows (from best to worst vascular reliability):

– Beneath the skin paddle (zone 1)
– On the surface of the muscle (zone 2)
– An extension anterior to the muscle (zone 3)
– An extension above the upper border of the muscle (zone 4)
– An extension distally above the iliac crest (zone 5)

The total area of this harvest is large: x cm by y cm (for example, $300 \, cm^2 \times 1 \, cm$ thickness will be $300 \, cm^3$) (Fig. 3.12a).

The additional adipose harvest should not produce a dissection that is anteriorly too wide between that

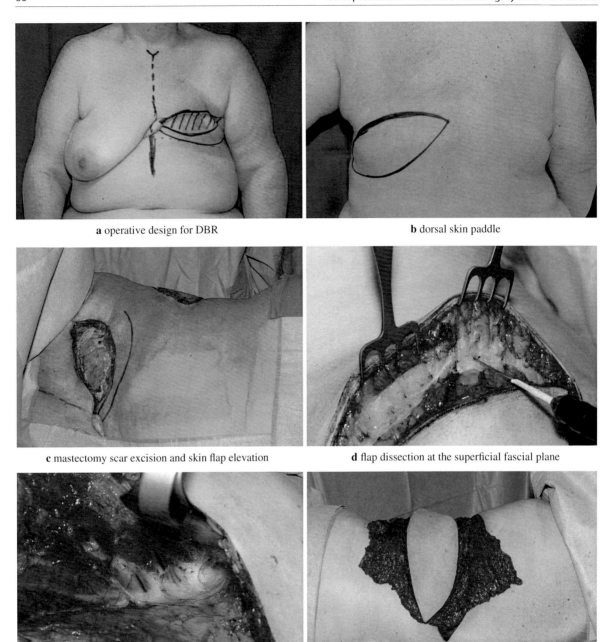

a operative design for DBR

b dorsal skin paddle

c mastectomy scar excision and skin flap elevation

d flap dissection at the superficial fascial plane

e thoracodorsal vascular pedicle on deep surface of flap

f flap harvested

Plate 3.11a–f Operative technique; autologous latissimus dorsi

dorsally and the area of mastectomy, in order to avoid the flap (with or without implant) slipping posteriorly into the donor area.

Harvesting of the upper fat beyond the superior border of the latissimus allows all of the fat anterior to the anterior border of trapezius and on top of teres to be included. This dissection is performed at the level of the perimysium of these muscles.

The distal fat harvest should collect as much volume as possible without being excessive, as this fat has

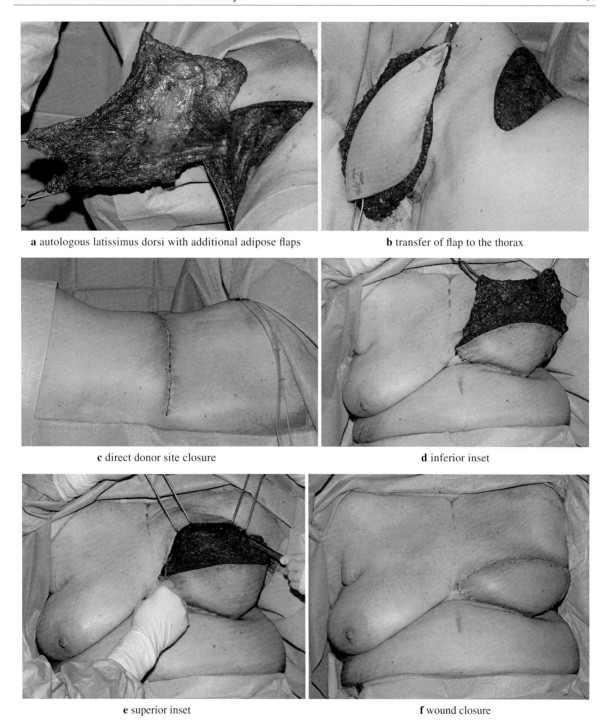

a autologous latissimus dorsi with additional adipose flaps

b transfer of flap to the thorax

c direct donor site closure

d inferior inset

e superior inset

f wound closure

Plate 3.12a–f Operative technique; autologous latissimus dorsi

the poorest vascularisation, and so may generate areas of fat necrosis and secondary depressions.

The muscle is then freed from distal to proximal along the deep surface. If there was any preoperative uncertainty over the integrity of the thoracodorsal pedicle, it must be identified as a priority (Fig. 3.11e).

The tendon of the muscle is then sectioned more or less completely. If complete, upon transferring the flap attention must be paid to ensure that the pedicle is not avulsed by undue traction. The tendon is subsequently attached to the thoracic wall.

After forming the tunnel, the flap is transferred onto the thorax and rotated 180° (Fig. 3.12b).

Second Stage: inset and modelling

This is done after closure of the dorsal wound, with the patient in a sitting position (Fig. 3.12d).

With immediate breast reconstruction and conservation of the breast skin, the flap is de-epithelialised and fixed to the pectoralis major muscle to obtain the desired shape. Usually the skin paddle of the latissimus remains as the area of the areola.

In other cases (secondary reconstruction or immediate reconstruction without skin-sparing mastectomy), the inframammary fold is marked and later fixed at a similar level to the other side. The inferior border of the skin paddle is inset as low as possible above the IMF to conceal the scar (Fig. 3.12d). The superior border is then sutured to the upper mastectomy flap with de-epithelialisation of a band of skin in order to improve superior quadrant filling. All of the distal extremity of the flap (which now lies uppermost because of the 180° rotation) is then folded back on itself and attached to the pectoralis major muscle beneath to give a tailored shape and volume (Fig. 3.12e, f).

Latissimus Dorsi Flap with Prosthesis

Flap harvest is performed in the same position as that described above for the autologous latissimus dorsi (Plates 3.13 and 3.14).

The incision may sometimes be vertical, which allows flap harvest in a supine position with a paravertebral bolster to avoid the need to change the patient's position, which is always time-consuming. This incision is generally restricted to thoracic coverage procedures rather than reconstruction. In general a skin paddle that closes directly is usually smaller and has less of an axillary dog ear during closure.

The surgical procedure is very similar to that of an autologous harvest (Fig 3.13a), but the skin flaps are raised on the superficial perimysium of the latis-

simus over its entire surface. Identification of the vertical muscle fibers of the anterior border is often easier more superiorly than inferiorly, where there is close intertwining with fibres of the external oblique. We harvest the maximal distal muscle possible, as it is this that fills the upper pole after rotation and flap transfer (Fig. 3.13a–c).

The muscle is raised from distal to proximal, taking care in the midline to avoid the trapezius (its fibres are oblique, unlike those of the latissimus, which are transverse) and superiorly with the serratus anterior. In fact, with the inferior border of the latter being free, it is easy to pass deep into the serratus and include it in the harvest.

The remainder of the dissection is identical to that described previously (Fig. 3.13c).

For flap modelling, the principles are identical. We prefer placement of the skin paddle in the mastectomy scar to optimise the quality of filling of segment 2 of the breast (Fig. 3.13e). The inferior border is placed as low as possible (Fig. 3.13f). Volume is obtained with a silicone prosthesis based on the form and dimensions of the contralateral breast and the patient's wishes (Fig. 3.14a). The inferior border is sutured in the IMF and the remainder of the muscle is spread out over all of the surface up to the supramammary crease. The prosthesis is thus completely covered with muscle (Fig. 3.14b). It is also possible to raise the pectoralis major and place the prosthesis beneath to give greater coverage of the superior pole (particularly in thin patients with thin muscles).

Special cases

In these cases, the skin paddle design may be either vertical with the patient positioned supine on a paravertebral bolster, horizontal or oblique with the standard decubitus lateral position. Harvesting is as described above (Fig. 3.15a–d) (Pousset 1986).

In certain patients, there is particularly obvious cutaneous laxity in the breast to be reconstructed (also an indication for implant-based reconstruction), but particularly thin tissues that would likely produce a poor result with implant alone. In such cases, one may offer reconstruction with a latissimus muscle-only flap to cover the prosthesis, or, alternatively, secondary fat transfer.

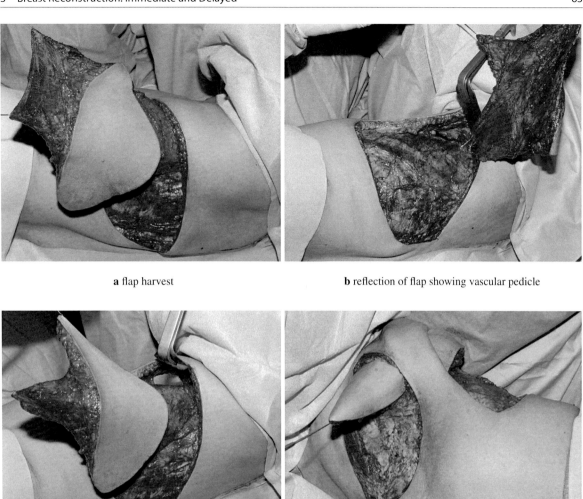

a flap harvest

b reflection of flap showing vascular pedicle

c dissection of tunnel

d passage of flap

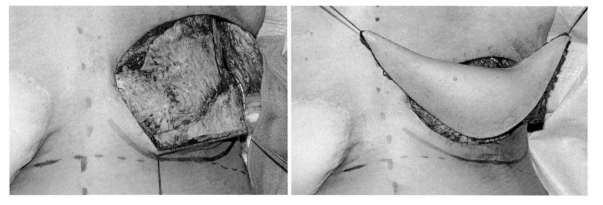

e preparation of recipient site

f inferior flap inset

Plate 3.13a–f Operative technique; latissimus dorsi with prosthesis

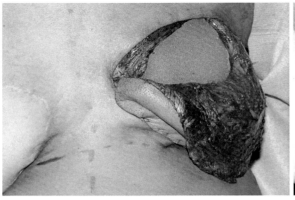

a prosthesis beneath pectoralis major

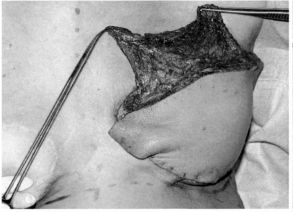

c superior pole covered by pectoralis and latissimus muscles

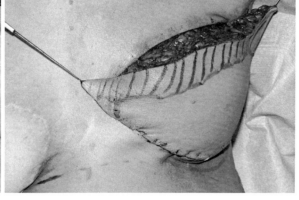

d design of deepithelialisation of upper part of flap

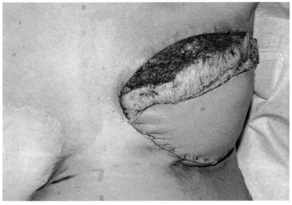

e deepithelialisation completed

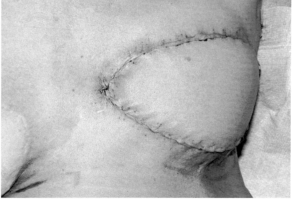

f flap inset

b suture of LD to pectoralis

Plate 3.14a–f Operative technique; latissimus dorsi with prosthesis: **a–f**

This harvest may be done without scars on the back, initially via an axillary scar (from axillary dissection if performed) for dissection of the pedicle and proxi-mal muscle and via the mastectomy for the remainder. Such dissection is assisted by either an endoscope or lighted retractor.

On occasion the latissimus muscle can be harvested without a skin island, through a short vertical incision beneath the axilla. If the thoracic skin envelope is of good quality, the muscle can be interposed between the envelope and the prosthesis to improve aesthetic results and risk of extrusion. This can be performed laparoscopically (Ramakrishnan et al. 1997).

Complications

Outside of the general complications of surgery, there are other, more specific, complications associated with this technique.

In a prospective series of 378 latissimus dorsi reconstructions, we observed:

– A haematoma rate of 3.2%.
– A lymphocoele rate of 28.3%. Notably, this complication was equally frequent in either autologous or implant-based reconstruction, but significantly higher for immediate (33%) compared to delayed (24%) procedures. This can be explained by the additional lymphocoeles at the mastectomy site. This number is probably underestimated, as many are drained percutaneously in the outpatient department and not always recorded.
– Skinecrosis of 1.8%. A higher rate of dorsal necrosis was seen in the autologous than in the implant group as a consequence of the more extensive dissection leading to ischaemia of the skin of the back. The thoracic necrosis rate was greater for immediate than delayed reconstructions, again due to the greater ischaemic risk produced by concomitant mastectomy.

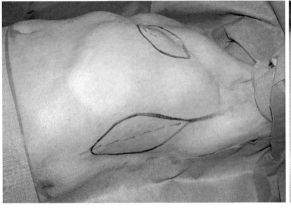

a operative design for coverage-only LD flap

b scar excision

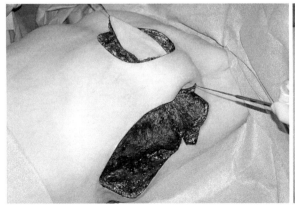

c flap raised and tunnelled

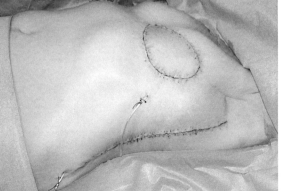

d wound closure

Plate 3.15a–d Latissimus dorsi flap for coverage

– Fever 1%, thrombosis 0.3%, and fat necrosis 1%. Vascular risk factors (obesity, smoking, etc.) in our series were not associated with an increased surgical risk.

Aesthetic sequelae of the dorsal scar are usually not of great concern to the patients, as are minimal functional consequences that allow a complete return to normal daily activities.

Conclusion

Breast reconstruction with the latissimus dorsi flap is a simple and reliable technique that gives results that are both superior to implants alone and more stable over time. With autologous flaps, the aesthetic results are stable over time, and close to those obtained with TRAMs. For implants, we observed a progressive deterioration of the results with time because of the adverse capsular contracture phenomenon and progressive ptosis of the contralateral breast.

There are relatively few complications and surgical sequelae compared with other techniques, making this technique one of the benchmarks in breast reconstruction.

Clinical results of latissimus dorsi flap breast reconstructions are presented in Plates 3.16, 3.17, 3.18 and 3.19.

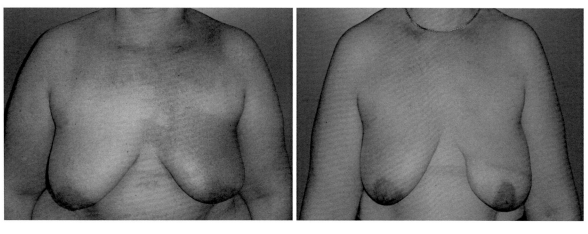

a left-sided cancer for mastectomy   **b** postoperative ALD and NAC reconstruction

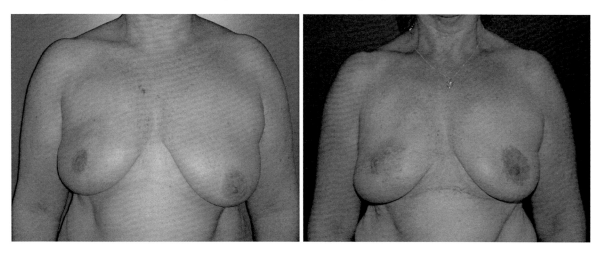

c right-sided cancer preoperatively   **d** postoperative ALD with NAC preservation

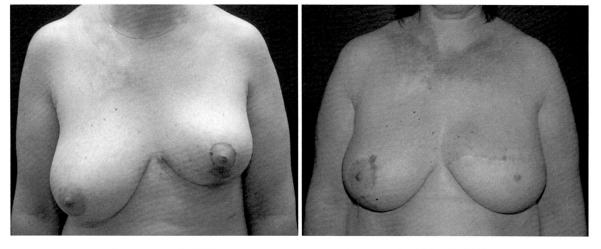

e previous unsuccessful BCT   **f** postoperative ALD with NAC reconstruction

Plate 3.16a–f   Immediate breast reconstruction by autologous latissimus dorsi flaps

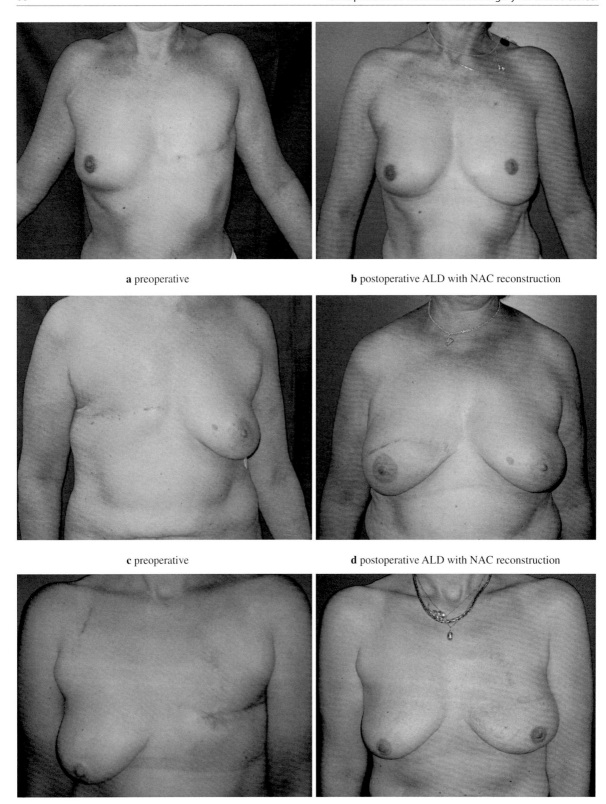

a preoperative   b postoperative ALD with NAC reconstruction

c preoperative   d postoperative ALD with NAC reconstruction

e preopeartive   f postoperative ALD with NAC reconstruction

Plate 3.17a–f   Delayed breast reconstruction by autologous latissimus dorsi (ALD) flaps

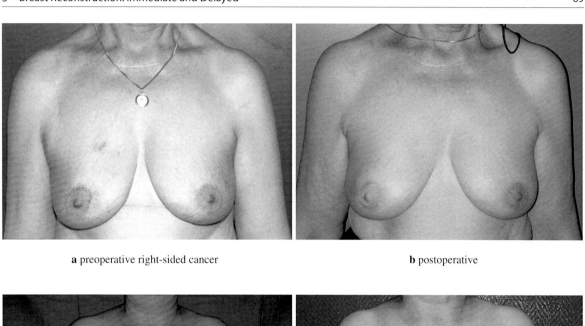

a preoperative right-sided cancer

b postoperative

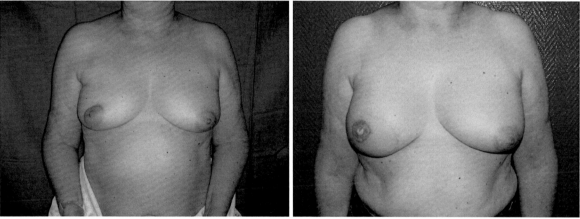

c preoperative right-sided cancer

d postoperative

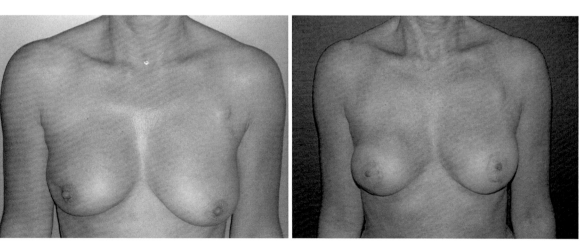

e preoperative with previous attempted BCT

f postoperative with symmetrisation

Plate 3.18a–f Immediate breast reconstruction by latissimus dorsi and implant

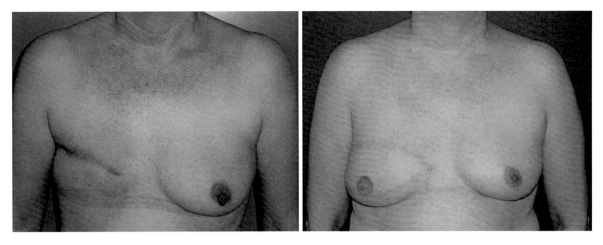

a preoperative   b postoperative LD-implant and NAC reconstruction

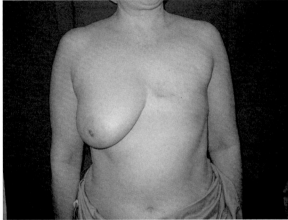
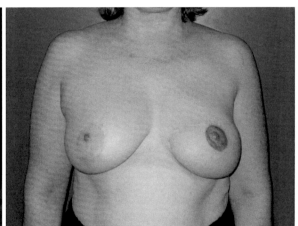

c preoperative   d postoperative LD-implant and NAC reconstruction with
                                                                                          symmetrisation

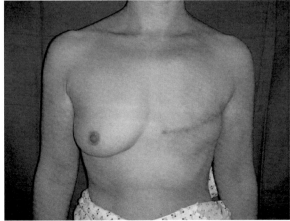
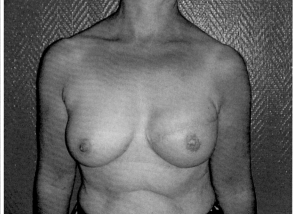

e preoperative   f postoperative LD-implant and NAC reconstruction

Plate 3.19a–f Delayed breast reconstruction by latissimus dorsi and implant

Transverse Rectus Abdominis Musculocutaneous (TRAM) Flap

Introduction

Described initially by Hartrampf in 1982, the TRAM is an autologous musculocutaneous flap that utilises the infraumbilical skin and fat, usually without a prosthesis, to reconstruct a breast after mastectomy in either an immediate or delayed fashion.

In contrast to the latissimus dorsi flap, here the muscle supplies limited volume, primarily vascular support.

Anatomical Review

The Rectus Abdominis Muscle

This constitutes, with the external oblique muscle, the anterior and superficial part of the abdominal wall (Caix 1999).

Each muscle is vertically orientated, with four bellies separated by three tendinous intersections, two above and one below the umbilicus. The intersections are adherent to the anterior and sometimes the posterior rectus sheath, which can make dissection difficult when separating the muscle from it. It originates from the fifth to seventh ribs and the xiphoid process and inserts into the pubic tubercle, bone and symphysis. The width narrows as it descends.

The rectus sheath comprises two leaves, anterior and posterior, resulting from the fusion of the anterior aponeuroses of the three lateral muscles (external and internal oblique and transversus). The two sheaths unite at the midline as the linea alba, but the posterior sheath is incomplete, stopping at approximately a quarter of its height at the arcuate line (line of Douglas). The posterior surface of the muscle is thus in contact with peritoneum at this point.

Vascularisation

The arterial supply of the abdominal wall is provided by a dual anastomotic network: one deep and muscular, the other superficial and adipocutaneous.

There are two arteries to the rectus abdominis muscle: the superior epigastric (a branch of the internal mammary) and the deep inferior epigastric (DIEA; arising from the external iliac artery). They anastomose within the muscle below the umbilicus.

The adipocutaneous arterial supply to the subumbilical abdominal wall is provided by musculocutaneous perforators. The most important are the three or four closest to the periumbilical midline. Their anastomosis, anterior to the superficial fascia, forms the subdermal plexus.

The venous drainage replicates the arterial network.

Functional Anatomy: The Flap Zones

There are four zones, I–IV, in order of decreasing vascular reliability of the adipocutaneous paddle. The closer to the pedicle, the better the arterial supply and perfusion pressure, and the better the venous return.

Classically, Hartrampf (1988) described the zones as follows:

- Zone I is the paramedian region beneath the umbilicus on the same side as the harvested muscle
- Zone II is the contralateral paramedian region
- Zone III is the homolateral outer region
- Zone IV is the contralateral outer region (Fig. 3.1)

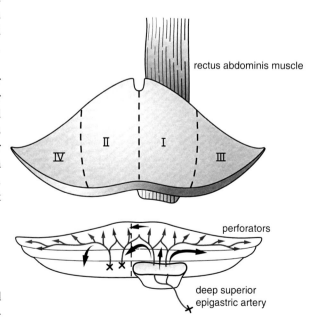

Fig. 3.1 Schematic of the TRAM and vascular zones

In the light of our experience, we have classified these four zones differently (Fig. 3.2).

Zones III and IV are of lesser vascular reliability, and so are excised in a bespoke fashion, confirming adequate blood supply.

Innervation

Innervation is provided by the lower six intercostal nerves. At least three must be sectioned for muscle paralysis.

These nerves, which accompany the intercostal arteries, penetrate the lateral border of the rectus sheath.

Functional Anatomy

The rectus abdominis muscles are strong ventral flexors and contribute very little to lateral inclination. Along with the oblique muscles, they are responsible for expiration, containment of the abdominal viscera and abdominal thrust, through increased abdominal pressure (for example micturition, evacuation and coughing). They also have a role in the global equilibrium of the ribs.

Operative Techniques

Unipedicled TRAM

We favour the harvesting of the muscle contralateral to the breast being reconstructed in order to minimise folding of the muscle carrying the flap. If necessary, the ipsilateral may be used.

The procedure demonstrated here (Figs. 3.3–3.25) is an immediate left breast reconstruction with a unipedicled right TRAM.

The design is made with the patient undressed, awake and standing (Fig. 3.3). It is then verified on sitting and lying down.

The markings are equivalent to those used in an abdominoplasty. The border of the upper abdominal incision is designed above the umbilicus. If the laxity of the abdominal wall appears insufficient, one can place the incision beneath the umbilicus, but this leaves an additional vertical scar.

The marking of the inferior border of the flap is usually made in the fold formed by the adipose apron, as low as possible above the pubis.

The lateral markings should allow dog ears to be avoided during closure. A low placement, close to the iliac spines, prevents elevation of the abdominal scar. A high placement guarantees the best vascular security of the cutaneous paddle, as it includes more periumbilical perforators.

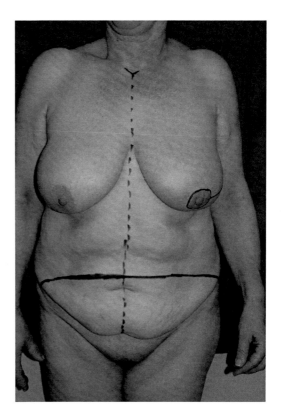

Fig. 3.3 Design with patient standing

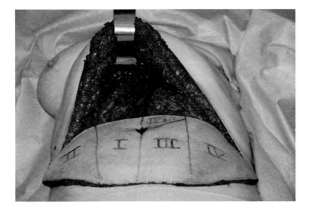

Fig. 3.2 Alternative vascular zones classification

For a DBR, the mastectomy scar is always excised for histopathological assessment and the mastectomy defect is recreated.

Incision of the Superior Margin and Elevation of the Superior Abdominal Wall

During this stage of the operation, two points are worth noting:

- Preservation of the fat above the umbilicus to avoid injuring periumbilical perforators
- Raising the upper flap at the level of the aponeurosis

Dissection should be wide: to the lower ribs on the side of muscle harvest and 2 cm below the future inframammary fold on the side of breast reconstruction (Fig. 3.4).

Incision of the Inferior Margin

This is done after verifying that the laxity of the abdominal wall allows tension-free closure (with the patient flexed at the hips) (Fig. 3.5). The lateral extremities of the incision are generously defatted to diminish the risk of excess fat and dog ears.

Raising the Adipocutaneous Paddle

This starts with the two lateral extremities of the flap at the fascial plane and proceeds medially to the perforators that mark the lateral limit of harvest of the infraumbilical aponeurosis (Fig. 3.6).

It is preferable to start by identifying the perforators on the contralateral side. They are not divided immediately, allowing their quality and distance in relation to the linea alba to be evaluated (Fig. 3.7).

The same manoeuvre is performed on the side of the harvested muscle. The principal perforators must be visualised without causing injury. Traction on the paddle must be gentle in order to avoid injury.

Freeing the Umbilicus

During this manoeuvre, it is important to preserve some periumbilical fat to avoid devascularisation of the umbilicus.

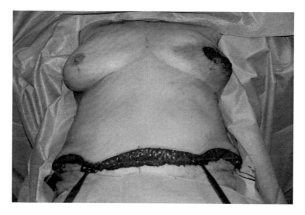

Fig. 3.5 Confirmation that closure is tension-free

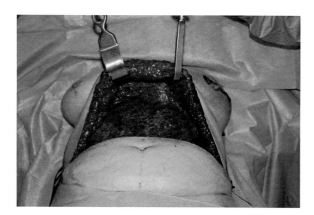

Fig. 3.4 Raising the abdominal apron

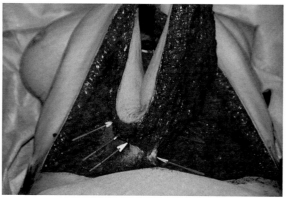

Fig. 3.6 The aponeurotic band is narrow and limited laterally by the perforators

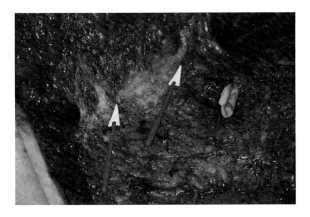

Fig. 3.7 Perforators are identified before section of the aponeurosis

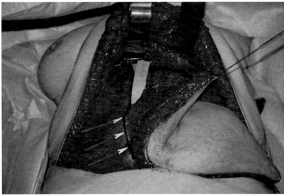

Fig. 3.8 The lateral limit is defined

Incision of the Aponeurosis and Freeing of the Muscle Borders

Supraumbilical

The lateral and medial borders of the rectus abdominis muscle are marked with ink (the width of the muscle varies from one patient to another), as are the costal margin, the xiphoid and the linea alba (Figs. 3.8 and 3.9).

1–2 cm of aponeurosis are preserved lateral to the midline to facilitate fascial closure.

The anterior fascial leaf is incised to preserve a small strip of central fascia, approximately 3–4 cm, on the anterior surface of the muscle that includes the perforators. The muscle is then freed from the fascia, from lateral to medial. The tendinous insertions are particularly adherent areas and care must be taken not to injure the fascia at this level (Fig. 3.10).

We do not preserve the lateral or medial muscular fibres because complete muscular atrophy occurs after division of the intercostal nerves.

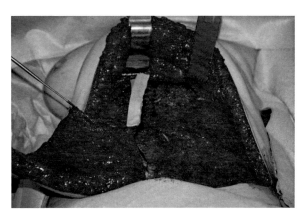

Fig. 3.9 The medial limit is defined

Infraumbilical

Laterally, the sheath is incised as close as possible to the perforators without damaging them, thus reducing the sheath harvest to the minimum and facilitating its subsequent closure.

Medially, after having sectioned the contralateral perforators and crossing the midline beneath the umbilicus, the sheath is incised at the level of the internal

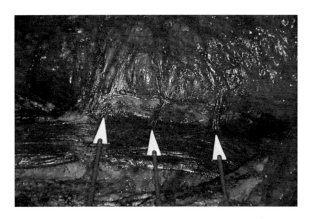

Fig. 3.10 The fascia is sectioned at the level of the perforators

perforators of the flap. It is usually possible to preserve 1–2 cm of sheath laterally without damaging the perforators as a result of diastasis (Fig. 3.7).

The medial and lateral sheath incisions meet each other at the inferior part of the harvested muscle.

Preparation and Division of the Deep Inferior Epigastric Pedicle

We habitually free the epigastric pedicle inferiorly at the level of the iliac vessels to yield the longest pedicle, in case a further vascular anastomosis (known as a turbo TRAM - see later) is required.

The inferior extremity of the rectus muscle is divided below the entry of the inferior epigastric pedicle.

Several sutures are used to attach the muscle to the sheath in order to minimise shearing movements and the risk of vascular damage to the perforators, which are fragile.

Resection of Poorly-vascularised Tissue

This is performed after division of the inferior epigastric pedicle and includes ZIV at least, usually with some part of ZIII also. In fact, such zones of poor vascularity must be sacrificed to ameliorate the perfusion of the remainder of the paddle. Its vitality is assessed by observing the bleeding at skin edges and the colour of the venous blood.

Elevation of the Flap

This step is performed in a completely paralysed patient (Fig. 3.12). The posterior surface of the muscle is progressively freed, from inferior to superior, and dissection is easy. One must take care to stay closer to the sheath than the muscle. Each intercostal and lumbar pedicle is ligated and divided as it is encountered (Fig. 3.13).

The eighth intercostal nerve is selectively divided at the inferior border of the lowest rib to facilitate muscular atrophy and limit traction on the pedicle during flap rotation. If the perforators are particularly closer to the umbilicus, the latter may be divided.

The superior epigastric pedicle is identified at the costal margin, emerging beneath the lowest rib close to the xiphoid, usually 2 or 3 cm from the midline (Fig. 3.14).

Division of the Upper Rectus Abdominis Muscle

This is done above the lowest rib to avoid injury to the pedicle on the deep surface. This manoeuvre allows optimal muscle atrophy in the perixiphoid region and

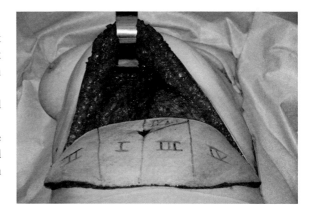

Fig. 3.11 The TRAM flap raised

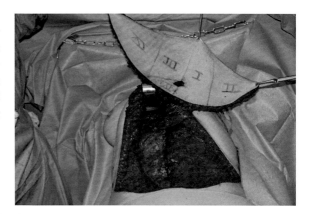

Fig. 3.12 Rotation of the flap

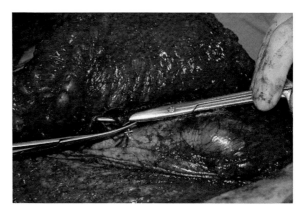

Fig. 3.13 Division of all intercostal pedicles

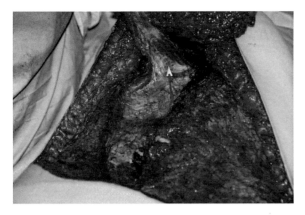

Fig. 3.14 Visualisation of the superior epigastric pedicle

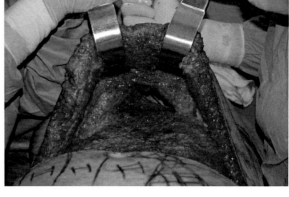

Fig. 3.17 A wide tunnel, particularly contralaterally

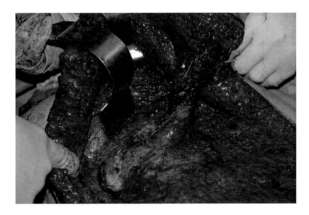

Fig. 3.15 Division of lateral part of muscle high on the lowest ribs

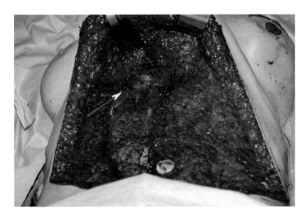

Fig. 3.16 Reduction of tension on the muscle as a result of lateral muscle division

facilitates rotation of the flap by transferring the pivot point more medially (Figs. 3.15 and 3.16).

Preparation of the Thoracic recipient site

Either the mastectomy scar is excised (in DBR) or mastectomy, with or without skin preservation, is performed (IBR). All specimens are sent for histopathological assessment. If a DBR is performed, the thoracic skin is raised widely medially and laterally as well as superiorly to the level of the clavicle. Inferiorly, the dissection is limited; in fact, the inframammary fold should be determined by progressive skin elevation in this area, with the patient semi-seated.

With IBR, once the mastectomy has been completed, a tunnel is created inferomedially, passing in part below the inferomedial contralateral breast, in front of the xiphoid and to the inferomedial part of the previous inframammary fold of the reconstructed breast. The dissection must be limited laterally to avoid lateral displacement of the flap.

Rotation and Passage of the Flap

Before the flap is passed through the tunnel, the width of the latter is verified; it must allow easy passage of the operator's hand.

The flap is then grasped by the lateral extent contralaterally and rotated through 180° (Figs. 3.12, 3.18 and 3.19).

This rotation shifts the lateral part of the flap to the axilla and the paraumbilical area to the medial angle of the future inframammary fold. The vascularity of the flap is assessed regularly at each stage.

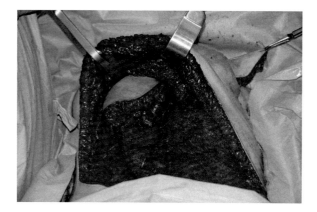

Fig. 3.18 Easy passage of the flap with no compression of the pedicle

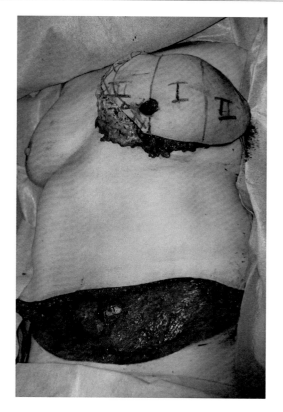

Fig. 3.20 Resection of zone IV and a variable part of zone III

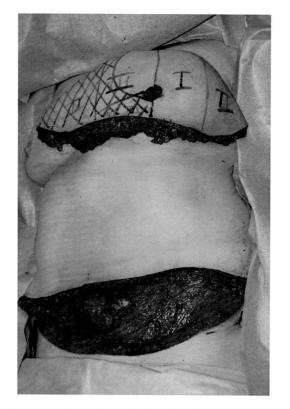

Fig. 3.19 180° rotation of the flap and marking of the zones to be excised

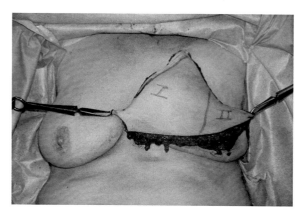

Fig. 3.21 Modelling of the flap on the thorax

Flap Modelling

The patient is placed in a sitting position. Rigorous evaluation of the viability of the flap allows appropriate resection of the lateral extremities (zones III and IV) (Figs. 3.20 and 3.21).

According to need, de-epithelialisation and burial of part of the skin paddle is performed. The flap is distributed to optimally occupy the volume between the infra- and supramammary folds. It is fixed deeply with interrupted sutures to the pectoralis major muscle. If not buried, the edges of the umbilicus are sutured together and make a small pleat at the inferomedial border of the new breast. A suction drain is inserted and the skin is closed in layers.

Abdominal Closure and Umbilical Reimplantation

The patient must be completely paralysed and lying down, but slightly flexed, during this part of the operation. In the majority of cases, a nonabsorbable mesh is placed deep into the anterior sheath and is completely covered when sutured. The mesh, when isolated in this way, reduces the potential risk of infection in the case of a postoperative seroma or delayed wound healing. The upper part of the sheath is closed as high as possible without causing compression of the pedicle (Fig. 3.24).

When the fascia may be closed without undue tension in thin patients, it may possible to manage without a mesh.

The umbilicus is "medialised" with several fixed points on the rectus sheath and then reimplanted in the midline. The skin is closed in two planes after the placement of two suction drains (Fig. 3.25).

Postoperative Protocol

The postoperative position aims to avoid pedicle compression and favour venous return. The patient is therefore nursed in a flexed-hip position with pillows beneath the knees to reduce tension on the abdominal

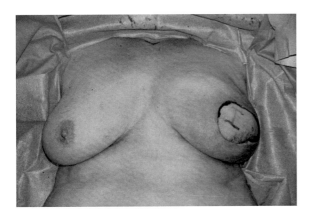

Fig. 3.22 Burial of the flap after deepithelialisation

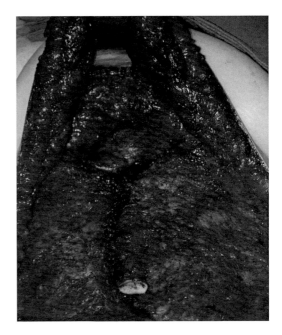

Fig. 3.24 Closure of the sheath with complete coverage of the mesh

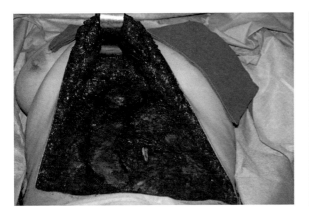

Fig. 3.23 Placement of the mesh into the rectus sheath

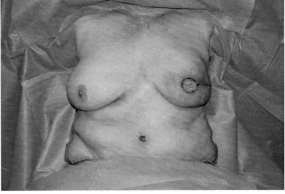

Fig. 3.25 Skin closure

wall. This position is maintained for 24–48 h according to the pain experienced by the patient.

The patient should be allowed out of bed on the first or second day if possible. Flap observations are performed every three hours for 10–12 h and then every six hours thereafter. Drains are removed after the second day (when the volume is < 30 ml per 24 h). A light diet may be commenced on the second day, progressing to a full diet at day three. A return to moderate sporting activities is allowed after approximately two months.

Other Techniques

Bipedicled TRAM

This involves harvesting both rectus abdominis muscles, and is used by some for improved vascular security (with the arterial supply being provided by both superior epigastric pedicles). It is therefore indicated for patients presenting with significant vascular risks (such as hypertension, diabetes and smoking).

This technique allows the harvesting of a wide cutaneous paddle with conservation of zones III and IV, and is particularly suited to the reconstruction of voluminous breasts (Wagner et al. 1991).

Positioning of the flap on the thoracic wall is more difficult because it must be rotated in the same way as an unipedicled TRAM, and so the two muscles overlap at the xiphoid process.

Abdominal closure is more difficult and mandates the use of mesh, so its complete coverage with rectus sheath is not always possible.

Harvesting both muscles increases both abdominal compression and postoperative pain.

Free TRAM Flap

This technique requires microsurgery so is more difficult than a unipedicled TRAM, but provides an improved vascular supply because the flap is vascularised by the DIEA. The latter is anastomosed to the thoracodorsal or internal mammary arteries. It is therefore preferable for high-risk patients: the obese, heavy smokers, and those with previous abdominal surgery and associated comorbidity.

On the other hand, it presents virtually the same donor site morbidity (rectus sheath harvest) as the pedicled TRAM.

Deep Inferior Epigastric Perforator (DIEP) Flap

The chief benefit here is the reduction in donor site morbidity, as only skin and fat is harvested, with the muscle and sheath being preserved.

Vascularisation is provided by perforators of the deep inferior epigastric artery.

Turbo TRAM

Harvesting is identical to an unipedicled TRAM, with the essential difference being the harvesting of the DIE vessels close to their iliac origin to provide additional length for a vascular anastomosis.

The DIE pedicle comprises two veins (which unite before joining the external iliac) and one artery. Microsurgical anastomosis is made to either the circumflex scapular vein and/or artery to preserve, if possible, the thoracodorsal pedicle. Usually vascular problems with the adipocutaneous paddle are secondary to venous return difficulties. This additional anastomosis ameliorates this problem. If the inflow is insufficient, one may similarly anastomose the DIEA to the circumflex scapular artery.

Indications for a turbo TRAM are thus similar to those for a bipedicled TRAM: enhancing the vascular supply to the skin paddle and allowing for a larger flap.

Discussion

Breast reconstruction, after mastectomy, by a TRAM flap is particularly well suited to women with wide, voluminous and ptotic breasts. It is sometimes used for smaller volume breasts when the patient declines the introduction of a foreign body, or if there is a deficit of thoracic tissue, or if the latter is thin and scarred (a contraindication to implant-based reconstruction).

Experience has also led us towards using a TRAM for the "conversion" of an implant-based reconstruction when complications, including delayed healing, extrusion of the prosthesis and adverse capsular contracture, occur. With disappointing aesthetic results, the prosthesis can also be replaced with a TRAM, bringing volume and good-quality skin. The results thus obtained are often highly satisfactory.

Finally, this flap may also serve as coverage for long-term complications of radiotherapy (radionecrosis), or for any oncological surgery (locally advanced cancer) that results in a wide thoracic wall defect. It has an occasional use for ASBCT Grade V (see chapter 5).

It is therefore indicated for a wide range of cases, and has proven valuable in numerous situations. However, it is also a technique not without risks and complications.

Advantages

Autologous breast reconstruction, without implants, results in a natural appearance and feel to the reconstructed breast. These results are durable over time and naturally reflect weight gain and ptosis, in addition to providing good symmetry with the contralateral side (only 33.9% required symmetrising surgery in our series, compared with 80% of implant reconstructions), since the texture and colour of the abdominal approximates that of the thoracic skin.

For the patient to benefit from this technique, she must present a suitable morphology: an infraumbilical pannus sufficient in proportion to the remaining breast, suitable skin laxity, and ideally no striae abdominalis.

Anterior abdominal scars are not an absolute contraindication for this technique, aside from subcostal scars, which are a source of abdominal wall necrosis. A midline infraumbilical scar mandates the sacrifice of half of the skin paddle, or the harvesting of a bipedicle TRAM. Pfannenstiel and appendicectomy incisions are not contraindications for this technique.

The TRAM may be used for delayed or immediate breast reconstruction (Granzow et al. 2006; Codner and Bostwich 1998; Miodrag and Milan 2001) (Fig. 3.26).

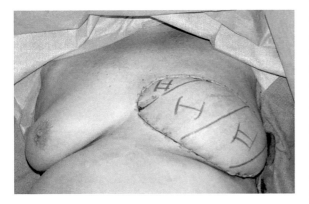

Fig. 3.26 Final flap inset showing vascular zones.

Our experience, as supported by the literature, shows that there is a real aesthetic advantage in TRAM reconstruction with irradiation, which may be done either before or after the reconstruction (Williams et al. 1995; Spear et al. 2005).

Disadvantages

The main disadvantage is the scar. As with all techniques that use a flap, TRAM reconstruction requires additional incisions compared to the use of an implant. However, a TRAM usually provides the secondary benefit of an abdominoplasty for those who select it.

It is not an operation devoid of complications of varying gravity. Some may require inconvenient prolonged wound care for the patient, but without significant future consequences for the flap and the quality of the reconstruction. Others are more worrying, risking the vitality of the patient or the flap. After analysing our series of 395 patients with TRAM reconstructions between 1991 and 2000 (Clough 2001b), we discovered the following.

The overall rate of complications is approximately 30%; these include necrosis (flap, abdominal wall), haematoma, lymphocoele, fever, delayed healing, pulmonary embolism, pain, bulges and hernia. These complications may be early (≤2 months) or late (>2 months).

Late complications comprise predominantly hernias and bulges, despite the routine use of prosthetic mesh. Residual abdominal pain in 20% and a reduction in muscular force in 36% (Lejour and Dome 1991; Mizgala et al. 1994; Futter 2000) have been reported.

Only 15% of the complications were considered serious in terms of revisional surgery required:

- Necrosis: >10% of the flap in 4.5%
- Abdominal necrosis and delayed healing: 2.5%
- Pulmonary embolism: 2%
- Hernias: 5%
- Mesh infection: 1%

These different complications are comparable, in number and gravity, to those encountered during autologous latissimus dorsi breast reconstruction (Delay et al. 1999).

In the literature, the risk of complications increases with obesity, anterior abdominal scars, and tobacco smoking. In our series, we found no statistical differences between these risks and our complications.

Unipedicle TRAM breast reconstruction is actually our preference now (65.3% of cases), with indications that have evolved with time: between 1991 and 1996 the most frequent techniques were uni- and bipedicle and turbo TRAMs. An analysis at that time showed there were more abdominal wall complications with a bipedicle TRAM. Because of this, free flaps and the DIEP were developed, the indications for such complex surgery ultimately being limited by the length and severity of the operative technique, which are little suited to our daily practice. They are best performed in specialist services that perform microsurgery on a daily basis.

Conclusion

TRAM flap reconstruction offers the advantages of an autologous reconstruction, particularly natural appearance and aesthetic results that remain stable over time as well as the secondary benefit of an abdominal improvement in the majority of candidates. It is not, however, free from complications, so many problems can be avoided (or at least reduced) with a good knowledge of the operative technique. Precise selection of patients in relation to their vascular risk allows the selection of a tailored technique after correction of the risk factors (smoking cessation, anticoagulation, diabetes control and so forth). Microsurgical techniques are a significant advance in the minimisation of abdominal morbidity, but are only performed by trained teams in specialist services. Results of TRAM flaps in IBR are presented in Plates 3.20 and 3.21, and DBR in Plates 3.22 and 3.23.

Free Flaps

Introduction

The 1970s saw the development of microsurgery, which then matured in the 1980s, resulting in an expansion of free autologous transplants with a multiplicity of indications (Arnez 1999). The principle of a free flap is the complete division of the artery and vein of its pedicle and their reattachment to recipient vessels (Figs. 3.27 and 3.28). This intervention requires the mastery of artery and vein suture techniques under the microscope or some other means of magnification.

Turbo TRAM

In TRAM flap breast reconstructions, the chief complication is adipocutaneous necrosis. Microsurgery allows the addition of vascular assistance to the flap.

During the raising of an unipedicled TRAM, the ipsilateral inferior epigastric pedicle (artery and vein) is dissected to its origin. If the flap shows signs of arterial, venous or mixed insufficiency at the end of the procedure, or some hours later, it is possible to salvage the flap with anastomosis of the DIE pedicle.

First, one must locate satisfactory recipient vessels: the external mammary vein or circumflex scapular pedicle, if not injured during previous axillary dissection. Unless in exceptional cases, we preserve the thoracodorsal pedicle for a subsequent latissimus dorsi flap if needed. The epigastric artery and/or vein are then anastomosed, usually under the microscope or with the loupes depending on vessel diameter (Figs. 3.29 and 3.30).

This simple manoeuvre allows the salvage of flaps that exhibit signs of insufficiency as long as it is done in the first few hours. Used at the time of TRAM reconstruction, it allows the use of a larger flap if the breast reconstruction is voluminous, but also minimises ischaemic complications in those patients with vascular risks

Free TRAM

The principle of this technique is to harvest only the rectus muscle that contains the musculocutaneous perforators. The aim is to minimise the abdominal wall sequelae from muscle harvesting. The inferior epigastric is dissected according to the same principles as used for vascular anastomoses. The pedicle will only be divided when one is certain that good quality recipient vessels are available. Some suggest that an end-to-side anastomosis to the axillary vessels should be made if required. Analyses of abdominal complications have not indicated any major benefit over the pedicled TRAM, probably because of the devascularisation and denervation of a significant proportion of the remaining muscle (Figs. 3.31and 3.32).

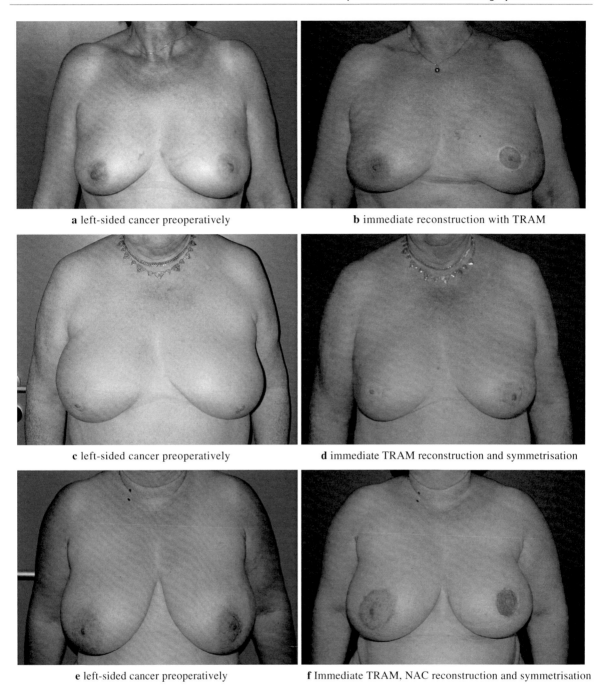

a left-sided cancer preoperatively

b immediate reconstruction with TRAM

c left-sided cancer preoperatively

d immediate TRAM reconstruction and symmetrisation

e left-sided cancer preoperatively

f Immediate TRAM, NAC reconstruction and symmetrisation

Plate 3.20a–f Immediate TRAM breast reconstructions—results

Deep Inferior Epigastric Perforator (DIEP) Flap

The first free TRAM flaps without muscle harvest appeared in the mid-1990s in response to the abdominal sequelae of free TRAMs (Blondeel 1999; Hamdi 1999).

The principle of this technique is dissection of the musculocutaneous perforators from their origin (inferior epigastric pedicle), through the muscle, and then to their entry into the fat (Heitman 2000). The remainder of the dissection (as well as the anastomoses) is identical to that of free TRAMs. Thus, no muscle is harvested

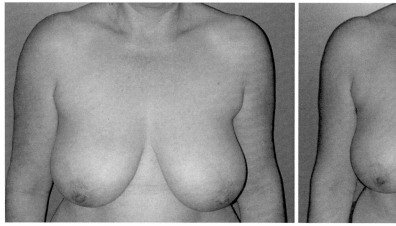

a left-sided cancer preoperatively

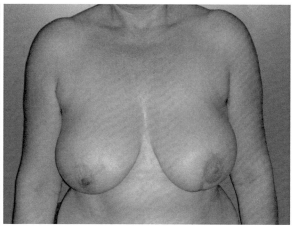

b immediate reconstruction post-TRAM

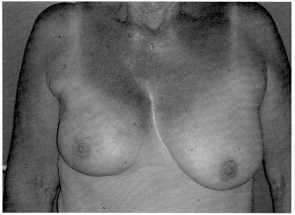

c left-sided cancer preoperatively

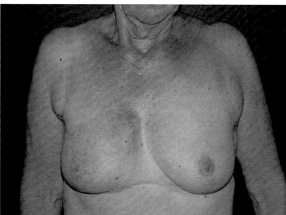

d postoperative TRAM after skin-sparing mastectomy

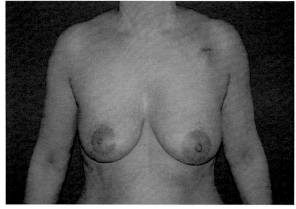

e bilateral preoperative

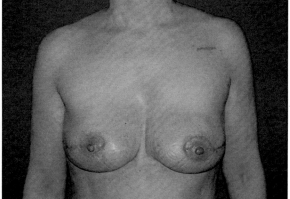

f bilateral TRAMs after skin- and NAC-sparing mastectomies

Plate 3.21a–f   Immediate TRAM breast reconstructions—results

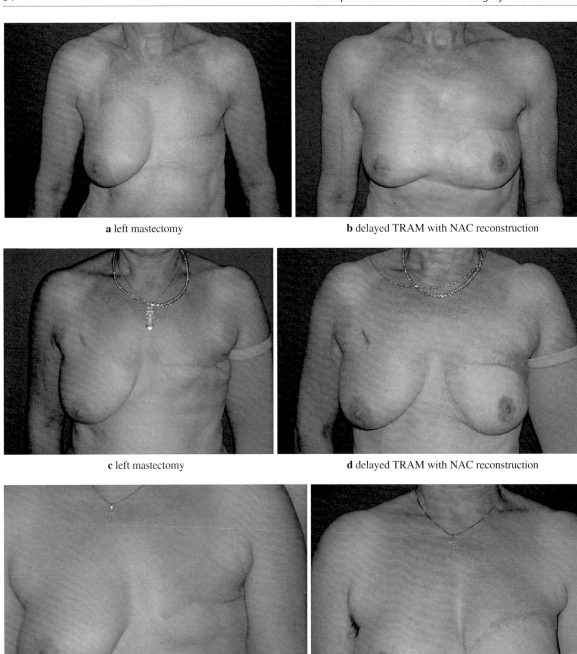

a left mastectomy   b delayed TRAM with NAC reconstruction

c left mastectomy   d delayed TRAM with NAC reconstruction

e failed implant-based reconstruction   f conversion to TRAM with NAC reconstruction

Plate 3.22a–f Delayed TRAM breast reconstructions

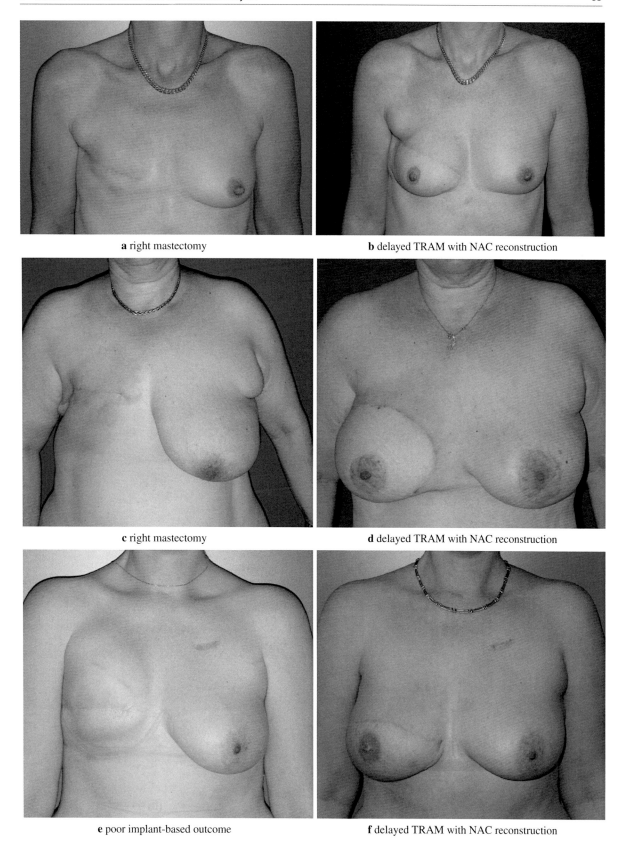

a right mastectomy

b delayed TRAM with NAC reconstruction

c right mastectomy

d delayed TRAM with NAC reconstruction

e poor implant-based outcome

f delayed TRAM with NAC reconstruction

Plate 3.23a–f   Delayed TRAM breast reconstructions

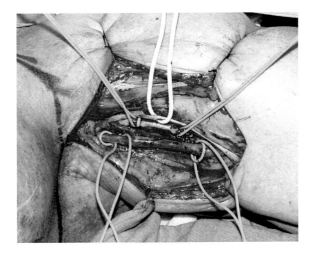

Fig. 3.27 Anastomosis—preparation of the vessels

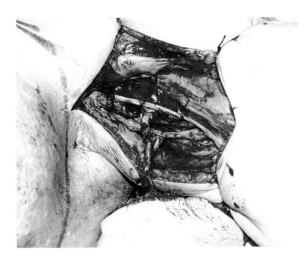

Fig. 3.28 Completed anastomosis

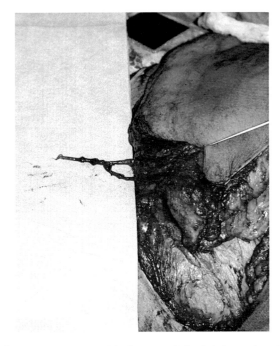

Fig. 3.29 Turbo TRAM—harvest of the inferior epigastric pedicle

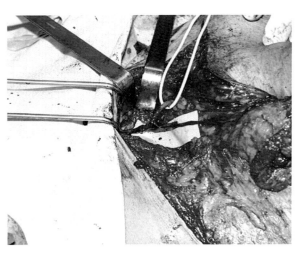

Fig. 3.30 Turbo TRAM—additional axillary anastomosis

in this dissection. The muscle is only partially devascularised and a useful innervation is preserved. The abdominal sequelae are thus extremely low (Keller 2001). However, the dissection is long and delicate and requires significant experience and a regular practice in vascular anastomoses (Figs. 3.33, 3.34 and 3.35).

Superficial Inferior Epigastric Perforator (SIEP) Flap

In rare instances, the dominant vascularisation of the abdominal wall comes from the superficial epigastric vessels (abdominal subcutaneous). One can therefore raise an abdominal adipocutaneous flap without any muscular dissection (Fig. 3.36).

Free Latissimus Dorsi

There are unusual circumstances where the only option for breast reconstruction is a free latissimus dorsi flap. In such instances, one may raise the contralateral latissimus

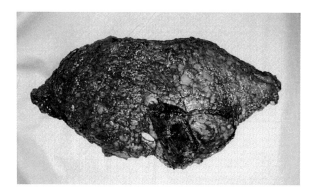

Fig. 3.31 Free TRAM with a muscule cuff

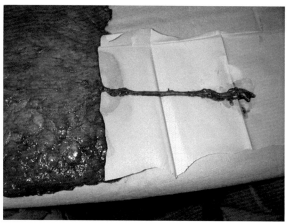

Fig. 3.34 Flap vascularised by the deep inferior epigastric artery and vein—DIEP

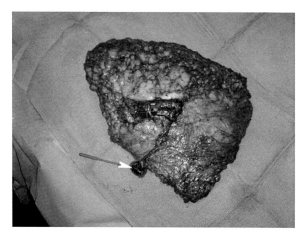

Fig. 3.32 Free TRAM with a long DIE pedicle

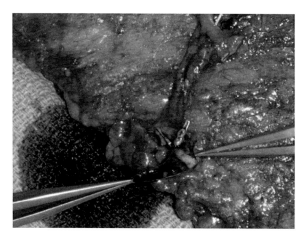

Fig. 3.33 Free TRAM—preparation of the vessels

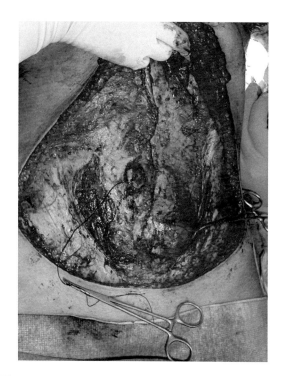

Fig. 3.35 Abdominal defect—TRAM (*right*) and DIEP (*left*)

sed to the recipient vessels (axillary, circumflex scapular, external or internal mammary) (Lanters 1997).

Gluteus

This flap is only used in breast reconstruction as a free flap. It allows reconstruction of the breast with skin

dorsi muscle and divide its pedicle close to the axillary vessels in order to provide vessels of a suitable diameter and a sufficient length. The pedicle is then reanastomo-

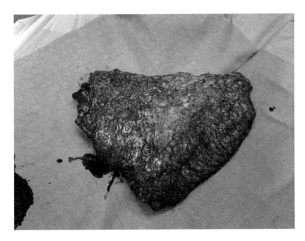

Fig. 3.36 Flap vascularised by the superficial epigastric artery and vein—SIEP

and fat from the buttocks. The donor site scar is often well concealed particularly if situated in the subgluteal crease (Paletta 1989). However, harvesting of this flap is a delicate procedure due to the vascular anatomy and requires ventral positioning of the patient. The indications are rare and require highly experienced teams.

Complications

Microsurgery presents additional complications compared to other techniques, particularly vascular anastomotic failure. There is a 2–10% risk of vascular thrombosis which, if re-exploration is not performed rapidly, leads to the loss (usually complete) of the reconstruction. Success rates depend on the experience of the teams, the vascular anatomy of the patients, and any previous radiotherapy. The risk of thrombosis can therefore rise to 15–20%. Thus, it requires teams that are trained and available to undertake surgical revisions without delay.

References

Arion HG (1965) Presentation d'une prothèse retromammaire. Com Rend Soc Fran Gyn 35:427–31
Arnez ZM, Khan U, Pogorelec D, et al. (1999) Rational selection of flaps from the abdomen in breast reconstruction to reduce donor site morbidity. Br J Plast Surg 52:351–4

Baker JL Jr, LeVier RR, Spielvogel DE (1982) Positive identification of silicone in human mammary capsular tissue. Plast Reconstr Surg 69:56–60
Bayati S, Seckel BR (1995) Inframammary crease ligament. Plast Reconstr Surg 95:501–8
Blondeel PN (1999) One hundred free DIEP flap breast reconstructions: a personal experience. Br J Plast Surg 52:104–11
Blondeel N, Vanderstraeten GG, Monstrey SJ, et al. (1997) The donor site morbidity of free DIEP flaps and free TRAM flaps for breast reconstruction. Br J Plast Surg 50:322–30
Boutros S, Kattash M, Wienfeld A, et al. (1998) The intradermal anatomy of the inframammary fold. Plast Reconstr Surg 102:1030–3
Caix P (1999) Anatomie de la paroi abdominale. Ann Chir Plast Esthet 44(4):289–311
Clough KB, Nos C, Salmon RJ, et al. (1995) Conservative treatment of breast cancers by mammaplasty and irradiation: a new approach to lower quadrant tumors. Plast Reconstr Surg 96:363–70
Clough KB, O'Donoghue JM, Fitoussi AD, et al. (2001a) Prospective evaluation of late cosmetic results following breast reconstruction: I. Implant reconstruction. Plast Reconstr Surg 107:1702–9
Clough KB, O'Donoghue JM, Fitoussi AD, Vlatos G, Falcou MC (2001b) Prospective evaluation of late cosmetic results following breast reconstruction: II. Tram flap reconstruction. Plast Reconstr Surg 107(7):1710–6
Clough KB, Thomas SS, Fitoussi AD, et al. (2004) Reconstruction after conservative treatment for breast cancer: cosmetic sequelae classification revisited. Plast Reconstr Surg 114:1743–53
Clough, KB, Sarfati I, Fitoussi A, et al. (2005) Reconstruction mammaire: résultats esthétiques tardifs des prothèses. Ann Chir Plast Esthet 50:560–74
Codner MA, Bostwich J 3rd. (1998) The delayed TRAM flap. Clin Plast Surg 25(2):183–9
Colic Miodrag M, Colic Milan M (2001) The use of pedicled tram flap for delayed breast reconstruction. Acta Chir Plast 43(1):7–10
Cronin TD (1963) Augmentation mammaplasty, a "new natural feel" prothesis. In: Third Int Congr of Plastic and Reconstructive Surgery, Amsterdam, 13–18 Oct 1963, p 41
Delay E, Jorquera F, Pasi P, Gratadour AC (1999) Autologous latissimus breast reconstruction in association with the abdominal advancement flap: a new refinement in breast reconstruction. Ann Plast Surg 42(1):67–75
Edgerton MT, McClary AR (1958) Augmentation mammaplasty; psychiatric implications and surgical indicatios (with special reference to use of the polyvinyl alcohol sponge Ivalon). Plast Reconstr Surg 21:279–305
Fitoussi AD, Couturaud B (2005) Evaluation des prothèses asymétriques en chirurgie d'augmentation mammaire. Ann Chir Plast Esthet 50:517–23
Fitoussi A, Couturaud B, Laki F, et al. (2005) Évaluation des prothèses asymétriques dans le cancer du sein. Ann Chir Plast Esthet 50:575–81
Futter CM, Webster MH, Hagen S, et al. (2000) A retrospective comparison of abdominal muscle strength following breast reconstruction with a free TRAM or DIEP flap. Br J Plast Surg 53:578–83

Granzow JW, Levine JL, Chiu ES, Allen RJ (2006) Breast reconstruction with the deep inferior epigastric perforator flap: history and an update on current technique. Plast Reconstr Aesthet Surg 59(6):571–9

Gui GP Tan SM, Faliakou EC, et al. (2003) Immediate breast reconstruction using biodimensional anatomical permanent expander implants: a prospective analysis of outcome and patient satisfaction. Plast Reconstr Surg 111:125–38; discussion 139–40

Hamdi M, Weiler-Mithoff EM, Webster MH (1999) Deep inferior epigastric perforator flap in breast reconstruction: experience with the first 50 flaps. Plast Reconstr Surg 103:86–95

Hartrampf CR Jr (1988) The transverse abdominal island flap for breast reconstruction. A 7-year experience. Clin Plast Surg 15(4):703–16.

Heitmann C, Felmerer G, Durmus C, et al. (2000) Anatomical features of perforator blood vessels in the deep inferior epigastric perforator flap. Br J Plast Surg 53:205–8

Henriksen TF, Fryzek JP, Holmich LR, et al. (2005) Surgical intervention and capsular contracture after breast augmentation: a prospective study of risk factors. Ann Plast Surg 54:343–51

Heymans O (2005) Smooth or textured implants: what to select? Ann Chir Plast Esthet 50:494–8

Janowsky EC, Kupper LL, Hulka BS (2000) Meta-analyses of the relation between silicone breast implants and the risk of connective-tissue diseases. N Engl J Med 342:781–90

Jenny H (1971) Areolar incision for augmentation mammaplasty. In: Fifth Int Congr of Plastic and Reconstructive Surgery, Melbourne, 22–26 Feb 1971

Keller A (2001) The deep inferior epigastric perforator free flap for breast reconstruction. Ann Plast Surg 46:474–9; discussion: 479–80

Lantieri L, Serra M, Dallaserra M, Baruch J (1997) Préservation du muscle en cas de reconstruction mammaire par lambeau libre de grand droit: du TRAM au DIEP. Note technique et résultats. Ann Chir Plast Esthet 42:156–9

Lejour M, Dome M (1991) Abdominal wall function after rectus abdominis transfer. Plast Reconstr Surg 87(6):1054–68

Lockwood TE (1991) Superficial fascial system (SFS) of the trunk and extremities: a new concept. Plast Reconstr Surg 87:1009–18

Maillard GF, Garey LJ (1987) An improved technique for immediate retropectoral reconstruction after subcutaneous mastectomy. Plast Reconstr Surg 80:396–408

Mathes SJ, Nahai F (1982) Clinical applications for muscle and musculocutaneous flaps. Mosby, St. Louis

Maxwell GP, Falcone PA (1992) Eighty-four consecutive breast reconstructions using a textured silicone tissue expander. Plast Reconstr Surg 89:1022–34; discussion 1035–6

May JW Jr, Attwood J, Bartlett S (1987) Staged use of soft-tissue expansion and lower thoracic advancement flap in breast reconstruction. Plast Reconstr Surg 79:272–7

Mizgala CL, Hartrampf CR Jr, Bennett GK (1994) Abdominal function after pedicled TRAM flap surgery. Clin Plast Surg 21(2):255–72

Muntan CD, Sundine MJ, Rink RD et al. (2000) Inframammary fold: a histologic reappraisal. Plast Reconstr Surg 105:549–6; discussion 557

Nava M, Quattrone P, Riggio E (1998) Focus on the breast fascial system: a new approach for inframammary fold reconstruction. Plast Reconstr Surg 102:1034–45

Nos C, Fitoussi A, Bourgeois D, et al. (1998) Conservative treatment of lower pole breast cancers by bilateral mammoplasty and radiotherapy. Eur J Surg Oncol 24:508–14

Paletta CE, Bostwick J 3rd, Nahai F (1989) The inferior gluteal free flap in breast reconstruction. Plast Reconstr Surg 84:875–83; discussion: 884–885

Pennisi VR (1977) Making a definite inframammary fold under a reconstructed breast. Plast Reconstr Surg 60:523–5

Pousset C, Salmon RJ, Soussaline M, et al. (1986) Utilisation du lambeau myocutané du grand dorsal pour les récidives du cancer du sein après irradiation. Ann Chir Plast Esthet 31:82–5

Ramakrishnan VV, Southern S, Villatane O (1977) Endoscopically assisted latissimus dorsi harvest and Prosthetic Placement. Br J Plast Surg 50: 219–20

Sergott TJ, Limoli JP, Baldwin CM, et al. (1986) Human adjuvant disease, possible autoimmune disease after silicone implantation: a review of the literature, case studies, and speculation for the future. Plast Reconstr Surg 78:104–14

Slavin SA, Colen SR (1990) Sixty consecutive breast reconstructions with the inflatable expander: a critical appraisal. Plast Reconstr Surg 86:910–9

Spear SL, Ducic I, Low M, Cuoco F (2005) The effect of radiation on pedicled TRAM flap breast reconstruction: outcomes and implications. Plast Reconstr Surg 115(1):84–95

van Nunen SA, Gatenby PA, Basten A (1982) Post-mammoplasty connective tissue disease. Arthritis Rheum 25:694–7

Wagner DS, Michelow BJ, Hartrampf CR Jr (1991) Double-pedicle TRAM flap for unilateral breast reconstruction. Plast Reconstr Surg 88(6):987–97

Wechselberger G, Del Frari B, Pulzl P, et al. (2003) Inframammary fold reconstruction with a deepithelialized skin flap. Ann Plast Surg 50:433–6

Williams JK, Bostwick J 3rd, Bried JT, Mackay G, Landry J, Benton J (1995) TRAM flap breast reconstruction after radiation treatment. Ann Surg 221(6):756–64; discussion 764–6

Omentoplasty or Kiricuta's Flap

The use of the greater omentum in breast cancer surgery was first described by Kiricuta in 1963.

The advantages of the greater omentum have been long recognised in numerous situations, including salvage of "at risk" intestinal anastomoses, tamponade of diffuse haemorrhage, particularly from the liver, and perineal defect restoration. It can also be used to pack fistulae, notably large vesicovaginal fistulae such as those seen in Africa.

Without dwelling on its complex embryology, the greater omentum is a richly vascularised structure that originates from the greater curvature of the stomach, between the right gastroepiploic vessels (from the hepatic artery), the gastroduodenal, and the left gastro-epiploics (from the splenic artery). The arterial circle begins at the anastomosis between these two systems, which constitutes the arterial supply of the greater curvature of the stomach. The greater omentum is vascularised by vessels that branch perpendicularly from the greater curvature. The greater omentum is thus richly vascularised by the two high-flow hepatic and splenic arteries and consequently presents a very low ischaemic risk, even with division of one of the afferent arteries.

There are also numerous anastomoses (visible by transillumination) between the two areas, which have no regular pattern.

Physiologically, the greater omentum is a "reserve" zone and so its volume varies widely between individuals. Actually, in northern latitude populations, it is generally voluminous and, contrary to what one might imagine, not comprised exclusively of fat. In fact, as with the peritoneum, it contains numerous lymphatics and a highly developed microvascular network. It is

this rich vascularisation that allows it to be used in plastic surgery, particularly in infected areas.

It is possible to release the greater omentum and use it as a flap for coverage of cases of substance loss in the anterior thoracic wall, and for many years its primary indication was the coverage of cutaneous radionecrosis.

To harvest this flap, a complete gastrocolic dissection must be performed, usually via laparotomy. It is acceptable to completely free the right and left angles of the omentum, visualising the second part of the duodenum to the right and the spleen to the left.

The dissection is by definition avascular, as it corresponds to the physiological adhesions of the gastric peritoneum and the transverse mesocolon in forming the gastrocolic ligament. The appearance of bleeding indicates that one has left the correct dissection plane! This dissection opens the cavity behind the omenta, which contains avascular adhesions that must be divided for correct mobilisation of the omentum. Also visible is the body of the pancreas in the depths of the greater sac.

According to the side and the site of placement of the omentum, one pedicularises the flap on one side or the other, generally contralaterally for thoracic reconstruction.

Ligatures must be placed between the arterial circle and the gastric wall. There is no risk of ischaemia to the gastric wall due to the rich and multiple intraparietal anastomoses.

Distally, the arterial circle must be carefully preserved in order to maintain a good vascular supply to the omentum. This dissection is not technically difficult, but must be done meticulously, and is a little lengthy on occasion because the omentum must be completely freed to allow its correct placement in the required area.

For thoracic coverage, the flap must be reflected superiorly and cross the abdominal wall en route to the thorax, where it is spread and attached. Surfaces of 300–1,500 cm^2 over areas 14–36 cm in height and 22–43 cm in width may thus be obtained.

Once positioned on the thorax, the omentum oozes abundantly and requires regular nursing care. It may be covered with a skin graft either at the time of flap harvest or some days later according to the surgeon's preference and the degree of cleanliness of the procedure. The graft typically does not "take" in its entirety at first, and a degree of secondary intention healing is the rule. A long-term failure of healing usually suggests the persistence of necrotic tissue, particularly bone.

Utilisation of the recently introduced vacuum-assisted closure (VAC) device may significantly shorten healing times (Ferron 2007).

The particular properties of the greater omentum allow it to be used to close infected and necrotic surfaces simply which renders this flap especially appealing when musculocutaneous flaps are either unavailable or being held in reserve.

However, the greater omentum may not be available, for example after excision, after its use in previous intestinal procedures and after cases of abdominal infection or trauma, so a careful history must be obtained from the patient. The patient's morphology is not a contraindication, and only extreme obesity or cachexia can pose technical problems.

Passage of the flap at the level of the xiphoid and/or costal margin constitutes a potentially weak area, with the risk of future herniation. Closure of the wall may be done without difficulty with a section of the omentum, which quickly acquires autonomous circulation.

Since 1993, it has been possible to harvest the greater omentum laparoscopically (Saltz 1993). This must be done by surgeons experienced in this technique and, according to the literature, the operative time is increased by about an hour, but modern techniques and instrumentation may well reduce this further. As with all laparoscopic surgery, abdominal scars are minimal, but the area of flap delivery and passage towards the recipient area leaves the risk of herniation as noted above.

The quality of the vessels of the omentum has led to its use as a free flap in certain cases; with well-trained teams, this can give excellent results. Despite the additional risks associated with microvascular anastomoses, it is worth remembering that abdominal wall closure is optimised and should not result in a risk of herniation.

Chauvet et al. (2006) recently published a breast reconstruction technique that uses the greater omentum. This is harvested as described above and then placed on the thorax following mastectomy. It is then modelled to form a volume compatible with the reconstructive requirement. Of course, this is only relevant in a few highly selective cases involving irradiated, well-informed patients with a particular morphology (small breasts, voluminous omentum) who are able to accept the risks of this technique and the eventual placement of a complementary implant.

Conclusion

The greater omental flap has lost a little of its notoriety because of significant developments with musculocutaneous flaps. The quality of this flap, its rich vascularisation, and its potential benefits in infected areas have made it indispensable to all those who manage breast cancer and it complications. At the boundary of intestinal surgery, oncological breast surgery and oncoplastic surgery, knowledge and use of this flap should be added to the armamentarium for breast cancer management.

Local Fasciocutaneous Flaps

Holmström Flap

Described in 1986 by Holmström (Pontes et al. 2006), this flap was then reported by numerous authors under the name of the lateral thoracodorsal flap (Lossing et al. 2001, 2000; Holmstrom and Lossing 1986).

We use it for tumours of the inferior pole in ptotic breasts, to avoid inverted-T scars, and for symmetrisation of a noncancerous breast (Plate 4.1).

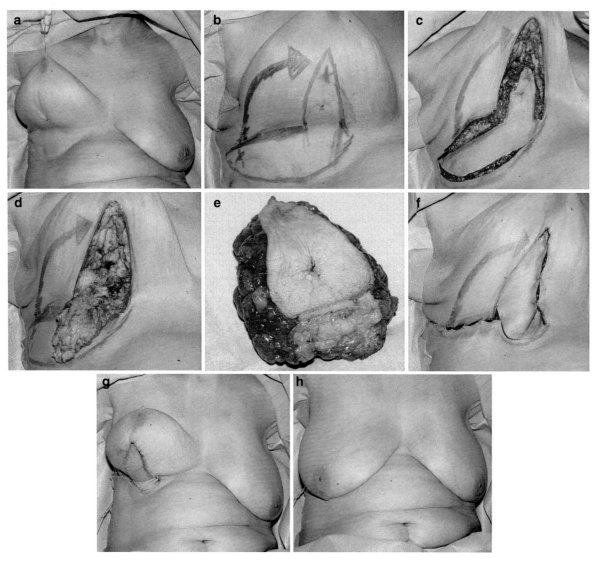

Plate 4.1 Holmström flap: operative technique: **a.** pre-operative right inferior pole tumour; **b.** operative design; **c.** incision of tumour and flap; **d.** tumour excision; **e.** operative specimen; **f.** flap rotated and donor site closed; **g.** flap inset; **h.** on-table result

A triangular excision is performed at the base of the breast in the inframammary fold, allowing a wide resection of the tumour. A triangle of a similar size, passing below the IMF with its apex directed laterally (Plate 4.1b), is then designed in segment IV of the treated breast.

The flap is raised progressively for at least 5 cm from the apex to the base, thus allowing it to rotate 90° with its apex towards the areola. The IMF donor site is closed directly (Plate 4.1f, g).

No procedure is generally necessary on the unaffected breast (Plate 4.1h).

Lateral Thoracodorsal Flap

This is a larger and more lateral fasciocutaneous flap derivative. It allows one, in certain cases, to avoid raising a more complex classical musculocutaneous flap for the patient.

High-quality results are obtained, particularly in older patients with sufficient subcutaneous tissue and good cutaneous laxity.

With an inferolateral base, the flap allows the breast shape to be recreated and a medium-volume implant to be placed for volume without further surgery.

The indications remain limited to particular cases, as with the Holmström flap.

The San Venero

Included here for historical completeness, the San Venero is a breast-sharing technique that is used when no other technique is available, or in very elderly patients with ptotic breasts. The aesthetic results are mediocre at best, because displacing the remaining breast towards the treated side displaces the NAC towards the centre, giving a "cyclops" appearance.

References

Chauvet MP, Giard S. Bonneterre J, Leblanc E (2006) Immediate breast reconstruction after total mastectomy using a laparoscopically-harvested greater omentum flap. In: San Antonio Breast Cancer Symp, San Antonio, TX, Dec 2006

Ferron G, Garrido I, Martel P et al. (2007) Combined laparoscopically harvested omental flap with meshed skin graft and vacuum-assisted closure for reconstruction of complex chest wall defects. Ann Plastic Surg 58:150–5

Holmström H, Lossing C (1986) The lateral thoracodorsal flap in breast reconstruction. Plast Reconstr Surg 77(6): 933–43

Kiricuta I (1963) L'utilisation du grand épiploon dans la chirurgie du cancer du sein. Press Med 71:15–7

Lossing C, Elander A, Gewalli et al. (2001) The lateral thoracodorsal flap in breast reconstruction: a long-term follow-up study. Scand J Plast Reconstr Surg Hand Surg 35(2): 183–92

Lossing C, Holmström H, Malm M et al. (2000) Clinical follow up of the lateral thoracodorsal flap in breast reconstruction: comparative evaluation from two plastic surgical centres. Scand J Plast Reconstr Surg Hand Surg 34(4): 331–8

Pontes R, Pontes GH, Serpa NP et al. (2006) Modified lateral thoracodorsal flap: a way out of a difficult problem. Aesthetic Plast Surg 30(5):633–4

Saltz R, Stowers R, Smith M, et al. (1993) Laparoscopically harvested omental free flap to cover a large soft tissue defect. Ann Surg 217:542–6

Introduction

Breast-conserving therapy (BCT) for breast cancer has become increasingly frequent since the 1960s. Today 60% of cases are appropriate for BCT, and some services have integrated "oncoplastic" techniques to allow conservation of the breast in up to three-quarters of cases.

The rising incidence of breast cancer, more than 40,000 cases annually (in France), increases the prevalence of adverse aesthetic results of breast conserving therapy (ASBCT). The rate of such sequelae remains stable at about 15–30% depending on the team, with at least 5–10% being significant, thus representing between 2,000 and 3,000 cases annually in France.

It is therefore essential to prevent such complications to avoid multiplying the number requiring—occasionally major—operative procedures in order to ameliorate these deformities.

Treatment of these sequelae is frequently complex as a consequence of the degree of deformity, and is particularly challenging when radiotherapy has been given.

There are some definitions of these deformities in the literature (Petit et al. 1989; Berrino et al. 1987, 1992; Slavin et al. 1992), and we have ourselves previously used a three-tier classification (Clough et al. 1998). The appearance of new surgical techniques and the evolution in our experience have stimulated the development of a revised five-level classification, which has been found to be better suited to the range of situations facing us.

Classification

Grade 1

This comprises minor malformations, generally resulting from a missed opportunity to remodel the gland at the time of BCT.

Although generally well accepted by patients, they occasionally prove problematic, particularly when located superomedially in the cleavage.

Techniques utilised in these situations include glandular rotation flaps for filling defects; these are always more difficult in irradiated areas. The appearance of autologous fat reinjection techniques (lipomodelage) has given us a simple treatment for such deformities. Long-term studies are, however, in progress to evaluate the benefits of management of grade 1 sequelae (see Chap. 7).

For minimally retracted radial scars, revision with debridement and Z-plasty is an alternative (Plate 5.1).

Grade 2

These are deformities of the treated breast which, as a result of surgery and radiotherapy, result in a diminution of both volume and natural ptosis (Plate 5.2).

Whilst an acceptable form is preserved, the volumetric asymmetry necessitates a procedure on the contralateral breast in order to match both the form and volume of the treated breast.

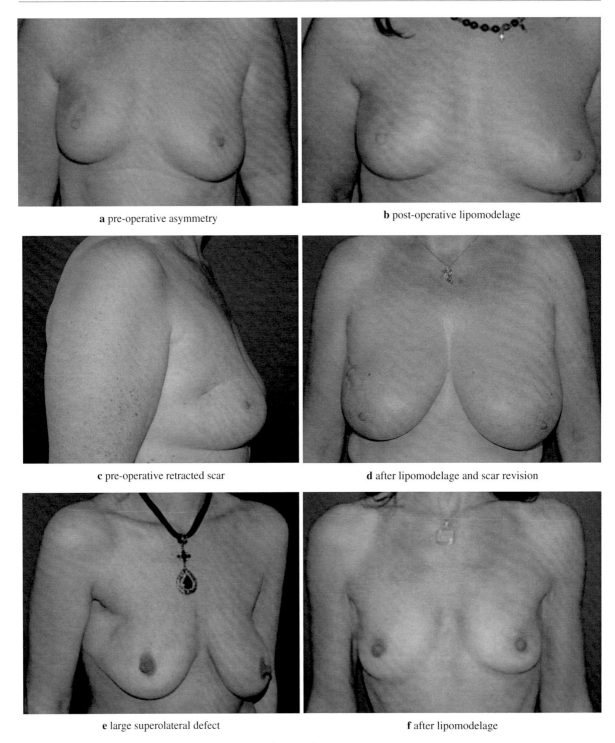

a pre-operative asymmetry   b post-operative lipomodelage

c pre-operative retracted scar   d after lipomodelage and scar revision

e large superolateral defect   f after lipomodelage

Plate 5.1 Aesthetic sequelae grade 1: lipomodelage and scar revision

Such anomalies are often simply managed with the application of various plastic surgical breast reduction techniques (see the section "Plastic surgical techniques in Breast Cancer surgery" in Chap.

2), allowing correction of asymmetry in the majority of cases.

Dimensions of the segments of the treated breast can be transferred to the opposite side for optimal

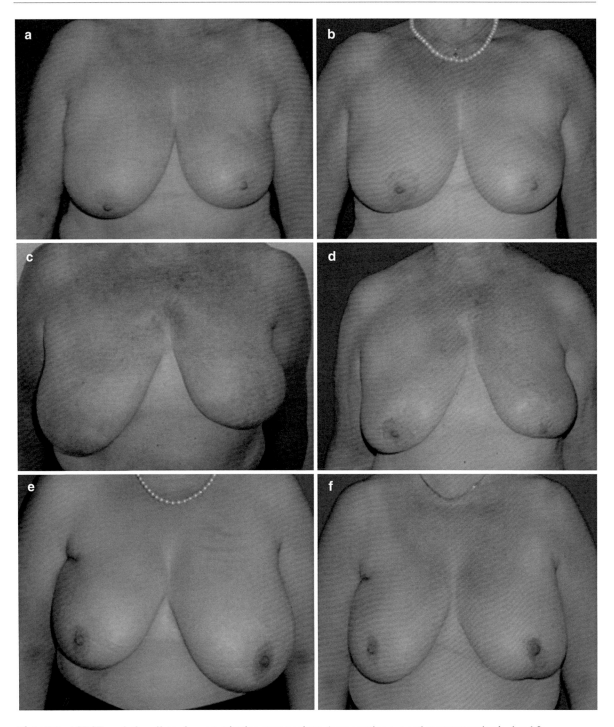

Plate 5.2   ASBCT grade 2: unilateral symmetrisation mammaplasty (preoperative a, c and e; postoperative b, d and f)

design purposes (Fig. 5.1). In particular, the ratios between segments I, II and III allows the planning of an areola of ideal size and position in proportion to the treated breast. Shortening segment III allows the best settling of ptosis in order to obtain optimal symmetry.

However, one must be aware of re-ptosis postoperatively in a breast that has not been irradiated. For this reason we generally overcorrect lightly.

For unilateral mammaplasty, the measurements are taken from the treated breast and transferred to the

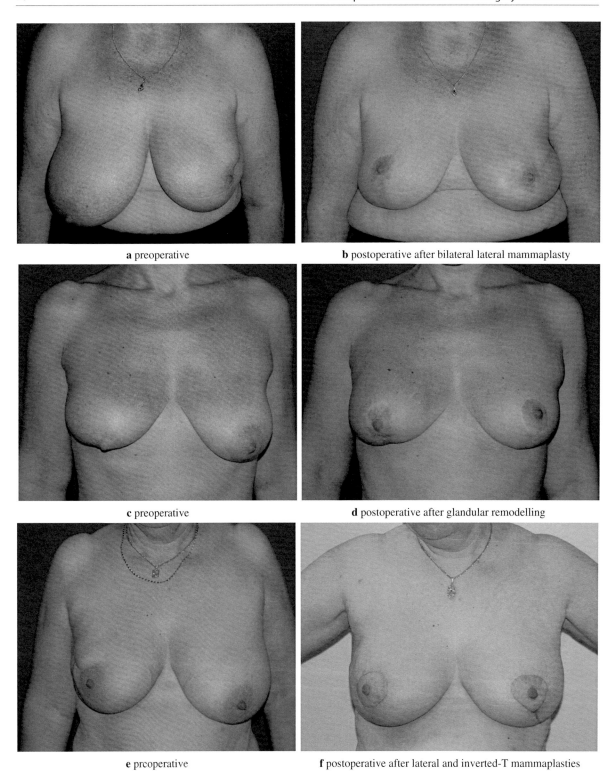

a preoperative

b postoperative after bilateral lateral mammaplasty

c preoperative

d postoperative after glandular remodelling

e preoperative

f postoperative after lateral and inverted-T mammaplasties

Plate 5.2a–f ASBCT grade 3; remodelling of the treated breast and symmetrisation as required

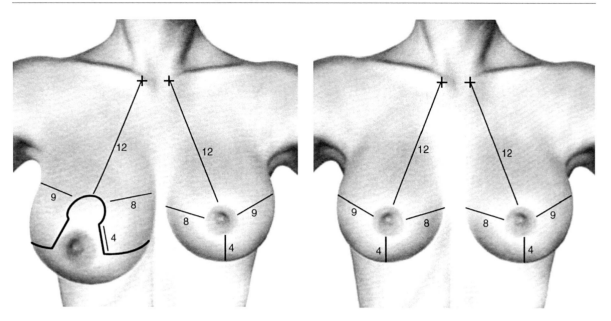

Fig. 5.1   ASBCT grade II: symmetrisation by carrying over the measurements from the treated breast

contra-lateral side. The measurements of the different segments as well as the areolar size should therefore be identical postoperatively (Fig 5.1).

Segments I and III will thus be diminished by 0.5–1 cm depending on the size and weight of the breast (see the section on plastic symmetrisation in Chap. 6).

Grade 3

With an asymmetry of the nontreated breast, these are similar to Grade 2 deformities, but the treated breast is not of a normal form and thus requires plastic surgical remodelling in order to improve it (Plates 5.3 and 5.4).

Such surgery is challenging in an irradiated breast, so it must be limited, particularly with respect to cutaneoglandular dissection. These interventions are generally limited to scar revisions with burying of fibrotic tissue. The NAC may require repositioning (usually lifting and centralising) or, on rare occasions, replacement as a full-thickness skin graft. Rarely, a mini-mal mammaplasty may be possible when irradiation has produced only minimal sequelae in the treated breast.

These gestures must be limited, as inflammatory reactions and the difficulties of wound healing on irradiated breasts are well known.

The nontreated breast may be symmetrised in the same fashion as ASBCT grade 2.

For very small volume breasts, the situation is different, as the opposite breast is usually flat with minimal ptosis. A bilateral augmentation with implants of differing volumes and projections is generally required with or without ptosis management of the contralateral breast with a periareolar technique (a vertical scar technique is sometimes used when ptosis is more marked) (Figs. 5.2a, b). Such cases are often very difficult because of the effects of radiotherapy, so the results may be unpredictable and are rarely entirely satisfactory. The patient must be informed of this before making an operative decision.

In certain intermediate cases, due to a major asymmetry, a reduction in the nontreated breast may be combined with an augmentation in the irradiated one; the complications, however, increase.

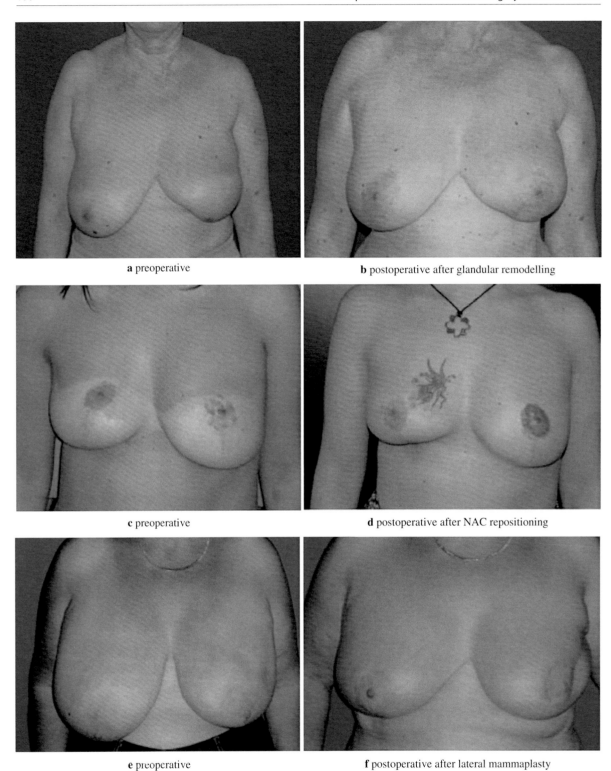

a preoperative

b postoperative after glandular remodelling

c preoperative

d postoperative after NAC repositioning

e preoperative

f postoperative after lateral mammaplasty

Plate 5.3a–f ASBCT grade 3; remodelling of the treated breast and symmetrisation as required

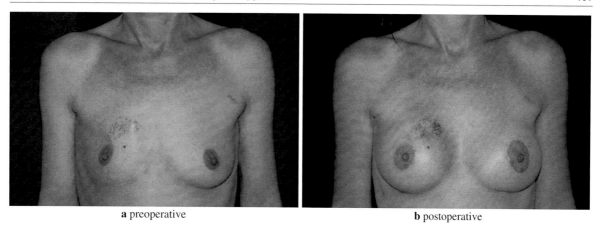

a preoperative   b postoperative

Plate 5.4   Insertion of asymmetrically projecting prostheses to achieve symmetry in the very small volume breast

Grade 4

As the classification proceeds, reflecting worsening deformity and thereby more difficult surgery, grade 4 deformities, as with grade 3, involve the treated breast, but are much more marked. As a result, remodelling of the breast is impossible due to the absence of a significant proportion of mammary volume, usually superolaterally or in the inferior quadrants. It is generally associated with a retracted and adherent scar, which requires wide resection to normal breast tissue (Plate 5.6).

Consequently, new tissue in the form of a musculocutaneous flap is necessary. An autologous latissimus dorsi flap is the most adaptable, but occasionally an abdominal flap may be used for extensive defects.

Depending on the result obtained with respect to form, ptosis and volume of the treated breast, reduction or remodelling of the contralateral breast may be required with mammaplasty using inverted-T, vertical or periareolar incisions (see ASBCT grade 3).

Grade 5

This group comprises major asymmetries where the treated breast is impossible to improve because of extensive fibrosis ("marble breast"). In such cases, the sole solution remains mastectomy and immediate reconstruction with either a latissimus dorsi (usually autologous) or a rectus abdominis flap, as reported in earlier chapters (Plates 5.7 and 5.8)

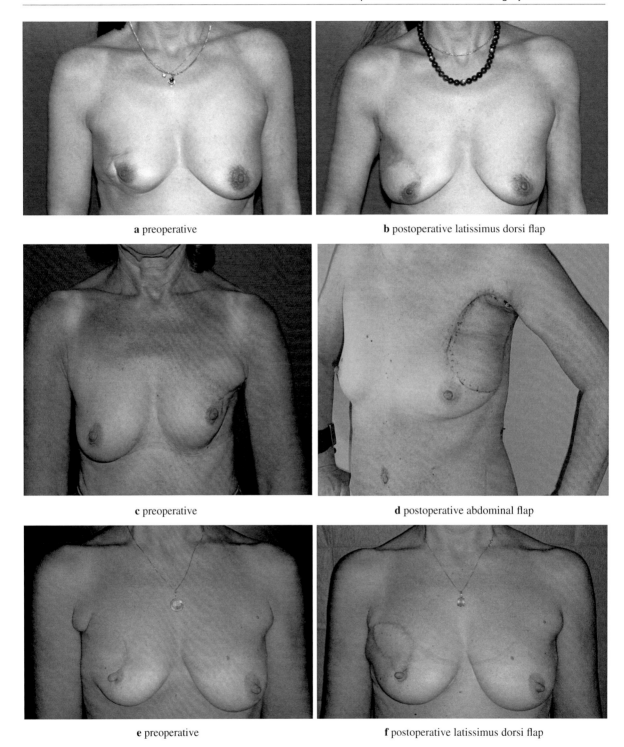

a preoperative

b postoperative latissimus dorsi flap

c preoperative

d postoperative abdominal flap

e preoperative

f postoperative latissimus dorsi flap

Plate 5.5.a–f ASBCT Grade 4: reparative surgery with musculocutaneous "patch" flaps

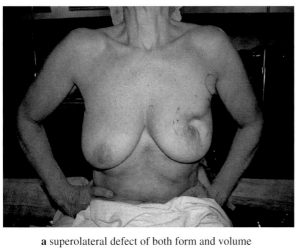

a superolateral defect of both form and volume

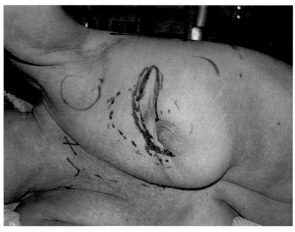

b lateral decubitus position

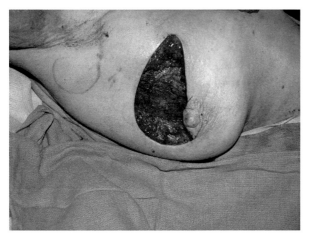

c actual size of defect after wide scar excision

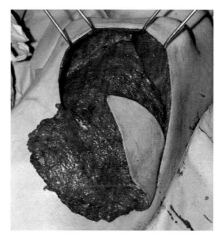

d harvesting of autologous latissimus dorsi flap

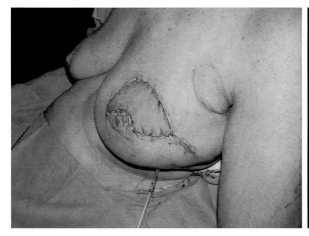

e flap inset

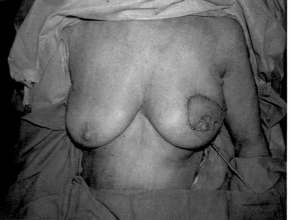

f on-table result

Plate 5.6a–f   ASBCT grade 4: operative sequence of autologous latissimus dorsi "patch" flap

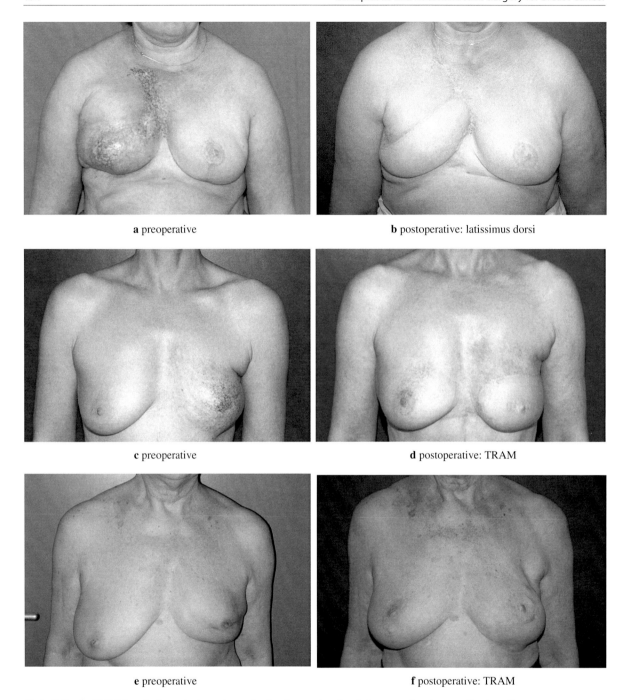

a preoperative

b postoperative: latissimus dorsi

c preoperative

d postoperative: TRAM

e preoperative

f postoperative: TRAM

Plate 5.7a–f ASBCT grade 5; mastectomy is required and reconstruction is by musculocutaneous flap transfer

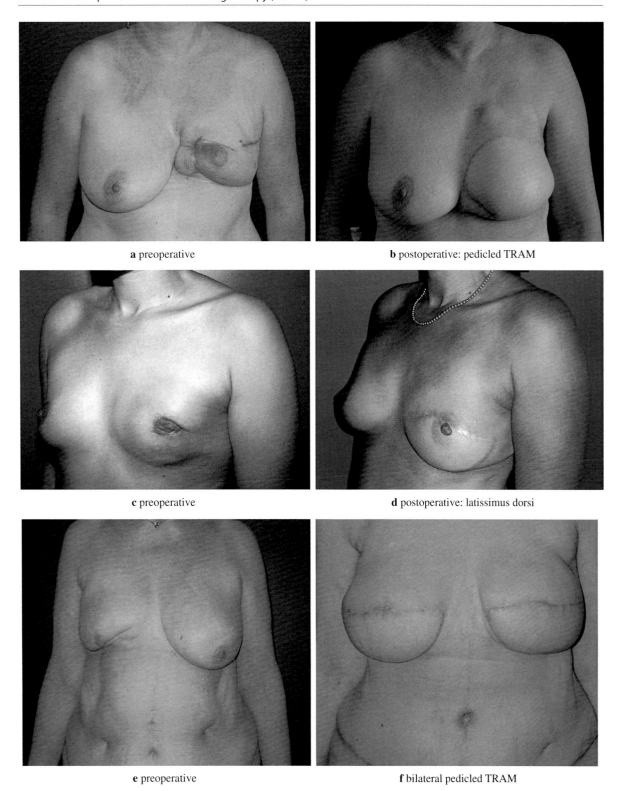

a preoperative

b postoperative: pedicled TRAM

c preoperative

d postoperative: latissimus dorsi

e preoperative

f bilateral pedicled TRAM

Plate 5.8a–f   ASBCT grade 5; mastectomy is required and reconstruction is by musculocutaneous flap transfer

Conclusion

This classification into five grades allows for the optimal categorisation of ASBCT according to progressive deformity and the surgical modifications necessary in the treated breast.

The treatment of these deformities is generally easier in grades 1 and 2, with simple procedures allowing symmetrisation of the irradiated breast.

In grades 3 and 4, the problem is more complex because remodelling irradiated breasts or interposing musculocutaneous flap is more complicated and not without significant complications. In grade 5, the complications are similar to other flaps, but there is the additional psychological burden of BCT failure. Awareness of potential aesthetic deformities assists with preventing and thereby reducing the incidence of ASBCT and its treatment, which may require major intervention.

Glandular plasties at a minimum and sometimes remodelling (see the "Mammaplasty for Breast Cancer"

section in Chap. 2) allow both the limitation of these complications and the facilitation of surveillance of treated breasts.

References

Berrino P, Campora E, Santi P (1987) Postquadrantectomy breast deformities: classification and techniques of surgical correction. Plast Reconstr Surg 79:567–72

Berrino P, Campora E, Leone S, et al. (1992) Correction of type II breast deformities following conservative cancer surgery. Plast Reconstr Surg 90:846–53

Clough KB, Cuminet J, Fitoussi A, et al. (1998) Cosmetic sequelae after conservative treatment for breast cancer: classification and results of surgical correction. Ann Plast Surg 41:471–81

Petit JY, Rigault L, Zekri A, et al. (1989) Poor esthetic results after conservative treatment of breast cancer. Techniques of partial breast reconstruction. Ann Chir Plast Esthet 34:103–8

Slavin SA, Love SM, Sadowsky NL (1992) Reconstruction of the radiated partial mastectomy defect with autogenous tissues. Plast Reconstr Surg 90:854–65

Reconstruction of the nipple–areola complex (NAC) is an essential part of the quality of a breast reconstruction. It should be possible to do this under local anaesthesia in order to both reduce the number of general anaesthetics and increase its acceptability.

Numerous techniques have been described in the literature (Amarante et al. 1994; Klatsky and Manson 1981; Eskenazi 1993; Anton and Hartrampf 1990; Kroll 1999; Weiss et al. 1989; Cronin et al. 1988; Little 1987; McCraw 1992; Brent and Bostwick 1977; Hallock and Altobelli 1993; Heitland et al. 2006). We describe the principal ones along with their advantages and disadvantages.

Patients are attentive to the form, colour and size of the areola, but also to the appearance and projection of the nipple. The combination of tattooing and a flap responds well to these demands.

Position and Form of the NAC

Matching the position of the areola with respect to the opposite side is essential for patients who will see themselves in a mirror. Whilst it can be done by eye, for optimal positioning we use measurements from anatomical landmarks including the midline, midclavicular line and the inframammary fold (Fig. 6.1).

We also use a novel technique for ideal positioning and areolar shape.

The periphery of the existing areola is outlined with a marker pen, and then traced onto paper. The tracing is cut out and placed in the optimal position on the reconstructed breast with a little adhesive or tape (Fig. 6.2).

This positioning must be made on a "stable" breast; in other words, some time (a minimum of two months)

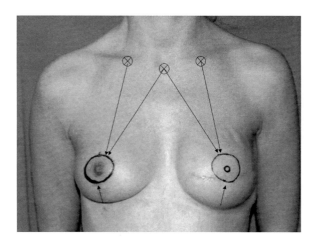

Fig. 6.1 The use of anatomical measurements for symmetrical placement of the NAC reconstruction

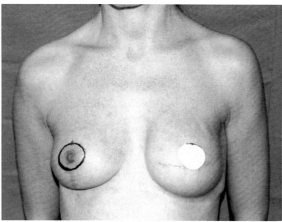

Fig. 6.2 Alternative method for positioning the NAC reconstruction

A. Fitoussi et al., *Oncoplastic and Reconstructive Surgery for Breast Cancer,*
DOI: 10.1007/978-3-642-00144-4_6, © Springer-Verlag Berlin Heidelberg 2009

after major glandular surgery. The combination of these two techniques allows optimal placement of the future NAC and compensates for any errors arising from measurements alone.

Areolar Reconstruction

The two most common techniques described for areolar reconstruction are:

– Tattooing
– Skin grafting

Tattooing

For the majority of cases we use unilateral tattooing if the colour is readily reproducible, and bilateral if the areolae are very pale.

It is generally a mix of two or three colours tattooed successively that best reproduces the irregularities of the existing areola and avoids a monochrome effect to the reconstruction. Experience is required to reproduce the existing colours as accurately as possible, considering that theatre lights, bleeding occasioned by the tattoo needle and vasoconstrictor effects in the anaesthetic influence perception of the tints.

If a graft is used to reconstruct the nipple, the areola is tattooed before inset. If a flap is used, only the future site of harvest is tattooed initially, the remainder being completed upon skin closure.

Skin Graft

Described by Little (1987), this comprises the harvesting of a full-thickness skin graft the size of the future areola, with the usual donor site being the inguinal crease.

De-epithelialisation of the recipient site gives a reliable base for the graft, which is affixed with interrupted, nonabsorbable sutures.

Note, however, that the graft tends to fade progressively with time.

Nipple Reconstruction

When volume allows, we use a contralateral nipple graft. In other cases we prefer a local flap, termed the "F flap".

Hemi-nipple Graft

For many authors, the autologous nipple graft is the technique of choice when possible (Georgiade et al. 1985; Millard 1972).

Harvesting can be performed in several different ways, depending on the form of the remaining nipple (hemi-section, summit, "cuneiform") (Figs. 6.3 and 6.4).

The contralateral neoareola is tattooed, and the recipient site de-epithelialised (Fig. 6.5). The nipple graft is harvested and attached with interrupted, nonabsorbable sutures in a tie-over dressing (Fig. 6.6).

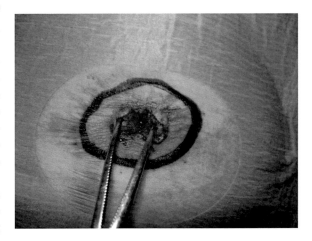

Fig. 6.3 Harvesting of the contralateral hemi-nipple

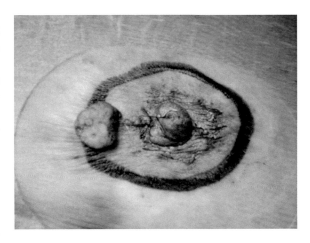

Fig. 6.4 Nipple graft and direct donor site closure

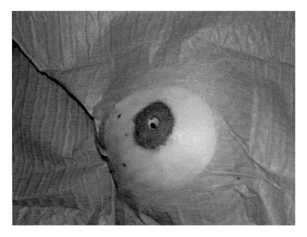

Fig. 6.5 Tattooing and de-epithelialisation of the recipient site

"F Flap"

When the contralateral nipple is too small or the patient refuses, or, of course, if there has been a contralateral cancer), we favour an adipocutaneous flap with two limbs that allows primary closure. Existing scars are used wherever possible (Figs. 6.7 and 6.8).

The technique involves raising two adipocutaneous flaps that are vascularised by a common central base then rolled, one into the other.

Depending on the size of the nipple to be reconstructed, the two limbs, often slightly asymmetrical, are measured as in Fig. 6.9.

After tattooing the selected area, elevation of the two flaps includes the full thickness of the skin and

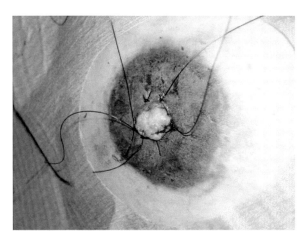

Fig. 6.6 Attachment of the nipple graft

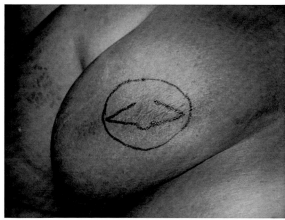

Fig. 6.7 Design for the F flap

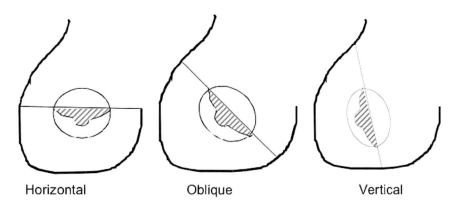

Horizontal   Oblique   Vertical

Fig. 6.8 Choice of incisions according to pre-existing scars

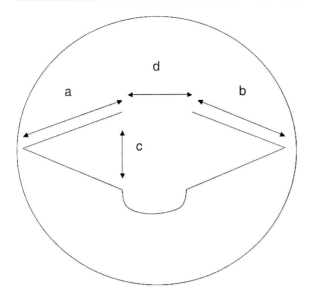

Fig. 6.9a–d Design for the "F flap": **a** 15–30 mm; **b** 12–25 mm; **c** 6–15 mm; **d** 15–25 mm (pedicle width)

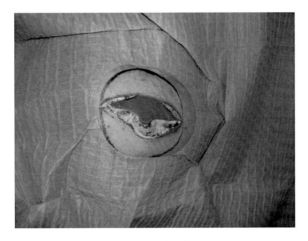

Fig. 6.10 Tattoo and elevation of the flaps

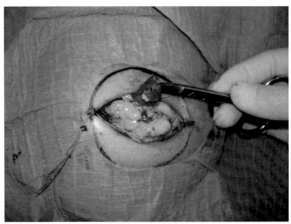

Fig. 6.11 Trial of optimal flap rotation

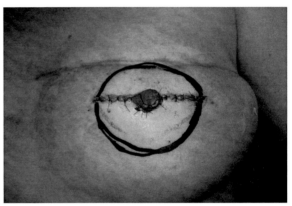

Fig. 6.12 Donor site closure and completed nipple reconstruction

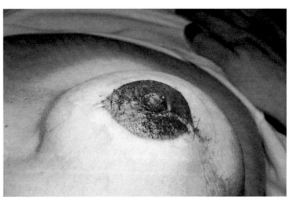

Fig. 6.13 Result at 2 weeks

subjacent adipose for augmentation of the nipple volume (Fig. 6.10). This volume is greater when the skin is thicker (as with the dorsal skin of a latissimus dorsi flap) and the result remains more stable.

The two limbs are raised, taking care with the pedicle of the flap. The limbs are subsequently crossed, one over the other, the longest generally being the more inferior, but both options are trialled to select the best (Fig. 6.11).

A deep, nonresorbable suture is placed at the deep surface of the two wings to give projection and prevent invagination of the neonipple.

It is often necessary to de-epithelialise a small area close to the neo-nipple, ensuring both a dermal bed and prevention of compression at the base.

Reconstruction of the nipple is then complete, so the donor site is closed. The areolar tracing is replaced and a new border outlined (Fig. 6.12). Further tattooing of the areas not previously included, due to distortion by the flap harvest, completes the areolar reconstruction (Fig. 6.13).

A thick, fenestrated tulle gras dressing is applied around the neo-nipple, followed by another layer. These are changed every two days and sutures are removed at 14 days, after which a simple dressing may be used.

We have reconstructed NACs with this technique since 1992 and have observed high-quality results that are relatively stable with time. The advantages of our technique include ease, speed and reproducibility. The resulting scar is limited.

"Z Flap"

This is a double-limbed flap, with each limb having its own separate pedicle (Fig. 6.14). Vascularisation is therefore more reliable and the risk of necrosis lower.

The position of the future areola is set and tattooed in the same fashion as for the F flap (Fig. 6.15).

The flap is designed so that the width of each pedicle and the distance between them are equal in diameter to the future nipple (Figs. 6.16 and 6.17).

The two flaps are raised full-thickness, as with the F flap, then sutured directly to each other with neither rolling nor plication (Figs. 6.18 and 6.19). Their thickness equates to half the reconstructed nipple.

For aesthetic reasons, it is useful to resect the tip of each flap in order to give a more natural appearance to the nipple (Fig. 6.20).

This new flap is employed if local conditions do not allow the F flap; notably where the skin is of not of high quality (Fig. 6.21).

Follow Up

If reconstruction fails (the nipple is either too small or flat), the same procedure can be performed again and

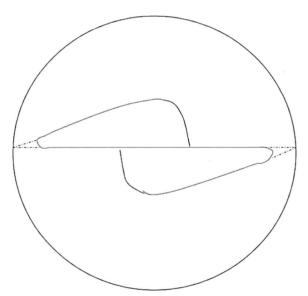

Fig. 6.14 Z flap

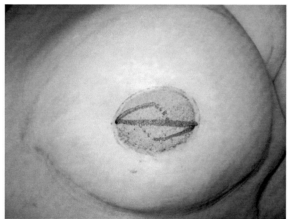

Fig. 6.16 Design of the Z flap

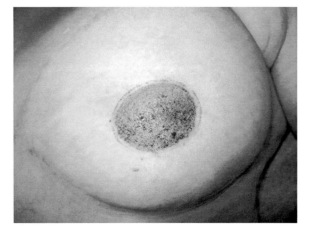

Fig. 6.15 Areolar tattooing

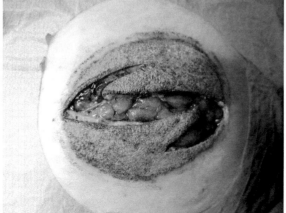

Fig. 6.17 Flap incision

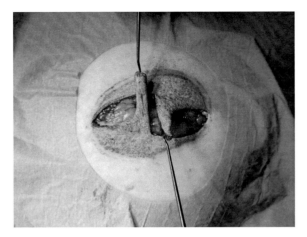

Fig. 6.18 Demonstration of the two flaps

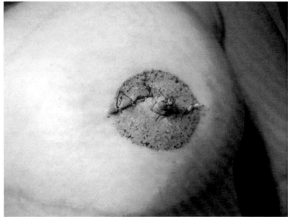

Fig. 6.21 Result at 2 weeks

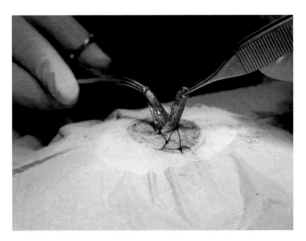

Fig. 6.19 Closure of the donor site

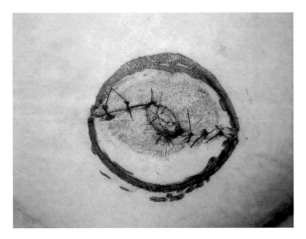

Fig. 6.20 Appearance after closure

advantage taken of the fibrosis occasioned by the initial intervention. The results are frequently improved.

Necrosis of one or other of the two wings is rare if the pedicle size is sufficient. In the long term, as with most such techniques, the areola fades progressively and nipple projection subsides, but an improvement in the result is almost always possible with a further procedure under local anaesthesia some years later, so this simple and reproducible technique is readily accepted by patients.

This technique frequently allows, particularly in implant-based reconstructions, utilisation of the mastectomy scar, whatever its orientation. In the case of a flap, when harvesting is central, the scar is limited to a line of 30–60 mm that is subsequently tattooed. This scar is certainly more easily closed than circular, inverted-T, S or H designs as used in other techniques.

Other Reconstructive Techniques

Distinction can be made between techniques utilising cutaneous flaps and others of grafted tissues. Others still are a combination of the two.

Flap Techniques

Since the early 1990s, skin flaps have allowed reliable nipple reconstruction.

Early techniques comprised skin plication (Little) or rolling ("snail"). Distinction can be made between those of either two or three limbs.

Little I and II: Areolar Graft with Local Flap

This is probably the earliest technique described and uses only autologous tissues (generally harvested from the inguinal area) for the future areola in association with a plicated skin flap at the recipient site.

The flap is designed and then raised after partial skin excision.

The graft is harvested, positioned with the nipple at its centre, then sutured in place (Plate 6.1).

It is very well known, probably because of its good reproducibility and lack of a need to tattoo, but distant donor sites are not always well accepted.

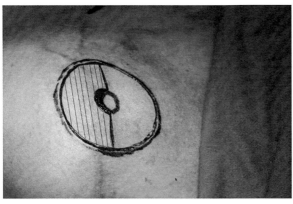

a design of flap

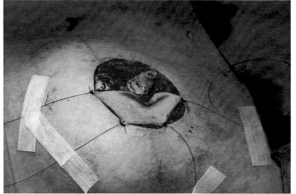

b positioning of graft

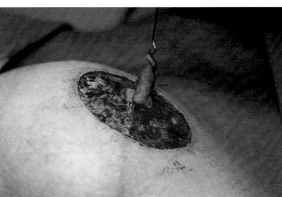

c raising of flap

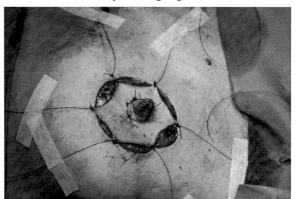

d appearance preclosure

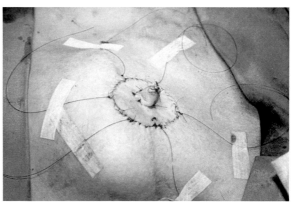

e neo-nipple

f on-table result

Plate 6.1a–f   Little's method of NAC reconstruction

However, long-term results are not particularly stable, explaining our reluctance to use this technique.

S Flap, Double Opposing Tab Flap, H Flap

The S flap is another early flap techniques described (Cronin et al. 1988; Weiss et al. 1989). Kroll et al. (1997) and Hallock and Altobelli (1993) developed variants based on the same concept of two identical and opposing flaps sutured to each other.

A circle centred on the position of the future nipple is designed, with a diameter equal to three times the nipple diameter.

An "S" or "H" is marked in the circle (Figs. 6.22 and 6.23), with the central line on the mastectomy scar. This creates two identical, opposing flaps that are raised and sutured to each other first by their bases and then by their edges. The skin graft is tailored (and therefore necessitates a de-epithelialisation of the recipient site).

The quality of the flaps is good, in addition to the projection, which remains stable over time.

Fishtail Flap

This is formed by rolling together two skin flaps with a common inferior pedicle so that the form evokes the tail fin of a fish (Figs. 6.24 and 6.25) (McCraw 1992).

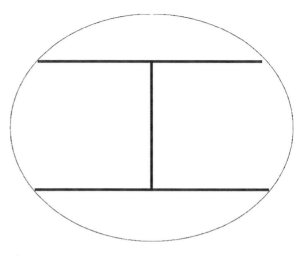

Fig. 6.23 H flap

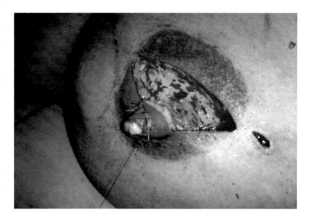

Fig. 6.24 Fishtail flap

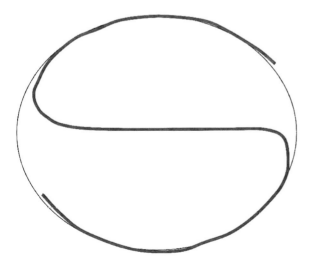

Fig. 6.22 S flap

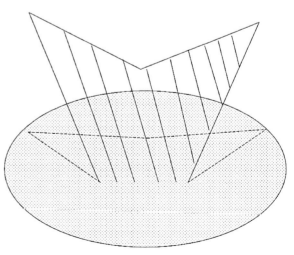

Fig. 6.25 Schematic of the fishtail flap

Star Flap

This technique is similar to the F flap and comprises three opposing flaps connected at their bases. It gives good results, but the donor site closure in a T risks delayed healing and skin ischaemia (Figs. 6.26 and 6.27) (Anton and Hartrampf 1990; modified by Eskenazi 1993).

C–V Flap

Described by Losken and Bostwick (2001), this is a bitriangular flap with a common base (the two Vs being identical in size), and with a third limb in the form of a C, the diameter of which is equal to the width of the V limbs and their "spacing". This third limb forms the superior part of the neonipple (Fig. 6.28).

Non-nipple Graft Techniques

Graft of Toe Pulp, Concha of Ear

Described by Amarante in (1994) then Klatsky (1981), the pulp of the second or fourth toe is harvested under local anaesthesia from a tracing that allows primary closure (Fig. 6.29), then grafted onto the recipient site. It tends to desquamate prior to the graft taking, but the aesthetic results are satisfactory for a limited cost (Heitland et al. 2006).

Conchal harvest is made through incision at the posterior surface of the pinna in order to be more aesthetic. The principle remains the same, but it is less well accepted by patients.

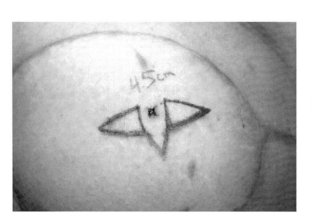

Fig. 6.26 Star flap design

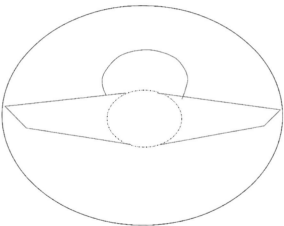

Fig 6.28 C–V flap

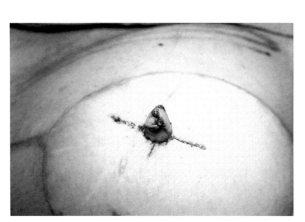

Fig. 6.27 On-table appearance of the star flap

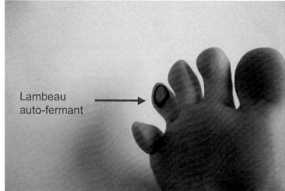

Fig. 6.29 Harvest of fourth toe pulp

Auricular or Costal Cartilage Graft

Associated with a full-thickness skin graft, these techniques augment nipple projection and are relatively easy to perform, but the donor site morbidity limits its their acceptability and widespread use (Brent and Bostwick 1977; Hobson et al. 1996).

Conclusion

In our service, 90% of patients undergoing a breast reconstruction will have NAC reconstruction. The preferred technique, F flaps and areolar tattooing, is simple, reliable and easily reproducible. It is always performed under local anaesthesia and does not require remote donor sites that often bother the patient. With particularly voluminous nipples, an autograft is possible.

With primary closure, this flap is our first choice, as it heals rapidly with a linear scar (often in the mastectomy scar) and produces good results.

Symmetrising Surgery

The aim of reconstruction is to match the size and shape of the contralateral breast to obtain a symmetry that is as close as possible to normal without the need to remodel. In the majority of cases, however, a contralateral symmetrisation is required due to contralateral natural ptosis that is difficult to achieve in the reconstructed breast.

All operative specimens should be sent for histopathological examination, as occult contralateral cancers are discovered in 1–3% (Staub 2008), which underlines the importance of systematic histopathological evaluation.

Symmetrisation by Prosthesis

When the reconstructed breast is either larger or better filled in segment II than the normal breast, a prosthesis may be offered that allows volume adjustment in addition to restitution of the shape of the superior hemisphere, which becomes progressively empty with time.

The principle is simple: a round silicone prosthesis with a projection adapted to the dimensions of the breast is generally used. We prefer a subglandular position, as the result is more natural and will age better. If the patient is very thin, the implant may be placed submuscularly.

If the breast to be symmetrised has been irradiated, the prosthesis is always placed beneath the pectoral muscle to reduce devascularisation of the gland.

The preferred incision is the IMF, but periareolar access may also be used. Rarely, we use an axillary approach. If the breast is ptotic, implant insertion is combined with mastopexy.

Augmentation–Mastopexy

When the contralateral breast is smaller and has a degree of ptosis that requires correction, we combine mastopexy, usually with a Lejour-type vertical pattern (Lejour 1994), with prosthesis placement. If the skin is not sufficiently elastic or the ptosis too great, an inverted-T skin excision (without glandular resection) may be used. The prosthesis is placed at the same operative sitting, ideally before the mastopexy order to best adjust the skin resection. We prefer a subglandular placement here also.

If the breast is of a similar volume, but ptosed, a mastopexy as described above is performed.

With an irradiated breast, augmentation with mastopexy but no glandular dissection is preferred. The risk of necrosis and adverse capsular contracture is higher and the patients must be well informed.

Breast Reduction

This consists of reducing and remodelling the nontreated breast to match that of the reconstructed breast. We utilise classical techniques, including those of Pitanguy (Piotti 1971; Lejour 1971), vertical scar and periareolar.

With irradiated breasts, we recommend particular caution because skin and gland elevation may lead to severe necrosis, which risks mastectomy in certain patients.

When Should Symmetrisation be Performed?

Contralateral breast symmetrisation is generally performed as a second stage. This allows retouching of the reconstructed breast, NAC and contralateral breast procedures in a single operation.

In certain circumstances, one may discuss immediate symmetrisation, particularly with delayed implant-based reconstructions. The contralateral breast is thus symmetrised at the same time, particularly when it is particularly hypertrophied or very ptotic.

When symmetrisation is planned for the same sitting as reconstruction, one should excise cautiously, as the definitive volume of the reconstruction frequently does not stabilise for several (usually 3–6) months, and so delayed symmetrisation is becoming more frequent.

References

Amarante JT, Santa-Comba A, Reis J, et al. (1994) Hallux pulp composite graft in nipple reconstruction. Aesthetic Plast Surg 18:299–300

Anton MA, Hartrampf CR (1990) Nipple reconstruction with the star flap. Plast Surg Forum 13:100

Brent B, Bostwick J (1977) Nipple-areola reconstruction with auricular tissues. Plast Reconstr Surg 60(3):353–61

Cronin ED, Humphreys DH, Ruiz-Razura A (1988) Nipple reconstruction: the S flap. Plast Reconstr Surg 81(5):783–7

Eskenazi L (1993) A one-stage nipple reconstruction with the "modified star" flap and immediate tattoo: a review of 100 cases. Plast Reconstr Surg 92(4):671–80

Georgiade GS, Riefkohl R, Georgiade NG (1985) To share or not to share. Ann Plast Surg 14(2):180–6

Hallock GG, Altobelli JA (1993) Cylindrical nipple reconstruction using an H flap. Ann Plast Surg 30(1):23–6

Heitland A, Markowicz M, Koellensperger E, et al. (2006) Long-term nipple shrinkage following augmentation by an autologous rib cartilage transplant in free DIEP-flaps. J Plast Reconstr Aesthet Surg 59:1063–7

Hobson MI, Williams N, Sharpe DT (1996) The "Mushroom" nipple-areolar reconstruction: a patient review. Ann Plast Surg 37(4):453

Klatsky SA, Manson PN (1981) Toe pulp free grafts in nipple reconstruction. Plast Reconstr Surg 68(2):245–8

Kroll SS (1999) Integrated breast mound reduction and nipple reconstruction with the wraparound flap. Plast Reconstr Surg 104(3):687–93

Kroll SS, Reece GP, Miller MJ, et al. (1997) Comparison of nipple projection with the modified double-opposing tab and star flaps. Plast Reconstr Surg 99(6):1602–5

Lejour M (1971) Indications de la méthode Aries-Pitanguy dans la ptose mammaire. Acta Chir Belg 70:5–10

Lejour M (1994) Vertical mammaplasty and liposuction of the breast. Plast Reconstr Surg 94:100–14

Little JW (1987) Nipple-areolar reconstruction. Adv Plast Reconstr Surg 43:7

Losken A, Mackay GJ, Bostwick J 3rd (2001) Nipple reconstruction using the C-V flap technique: a long-term evaluation. Plast Reconstr Surg 108(2):1602–5

McCraw JB (1992) "Fish-tailed flap" for nipple reconstruction. Aesthetic and Reconstructive Surgery of the Breast Symposium sponsored by Manhatten Eye, Ear and Throat Hospital

Millard DR Jr (1972) Nipple and areola reconstruction by split-skin graft from the normal side. Plast Reconstr Surg 50(4):350–3

Piotti F (1971) Mastoplasty by the Pitanguy method. Minerva Chir 26:173–85

Staub G, Fitoussi A, Falcou M-C, Salmon RJ (2008) Breast cancer surgery: use of mammaplasty. Results. Series of 298 cases. Ann Chir Plast Esthet 53:124–34

Weiss J, Herman O, Rosenberg L, et al. (1989) The S nipple-areola reconstruction. Plast Reconstr Surg 83(5):904–6

Lipomodelage and Breast Surgery

7

Historical Background

Lipomodelage, or fat transfer, is essentially an adipose tissue autograft that is used in both aesthetic and reconstructive surgery to correct volumetric defects.

For over a century (Mojallal and Foyatier 2004) surgeons have attempted to reconstruct or augment the volume of breasts using autogenous fat. The early 1980s saw the development of liposuction, which prompted the use of this unpurified fat by-product in breast surgery (Illouz 1986; Fournier 1985): fat transfer was thus created.

Following the work of Colemen et al. (1994), autologous adipocyte grafting has been refined so that purified fat, harvested by an atraumatic technique, is now the current standard.

Technique

The principle of this technique is to be as atraumatic as possible: the fat must be neither compressed nor filtered nor washed nor aspirated or reinjected under high pressure, nor mixed with other blood constituents nor frozen. These precise rules aim at obtaining the most stable and best quality results over time (Société Française de Chirurgie Plastique Reconstructrice et Esthétique 2004).

It may be performed under either general or local anaesthesia; however, any injection into the operative site must not damage the adipocytes. Whilst Lidocaine (Xylocaine) appears not to have any deleterious effects, the situation for adrenaline remains equivocal.

Fat Harvesting

This is done ideally without preliminary infiltration, using low-pressure liposuction, which is less traumatic than surgical harvesting and has replaced it (Sinna et al. 2006). Manual harvest using a syringe allows a better yield of adipocytes compared to that performed under pressure (Figs. 7.1–7.3).

According to Coleman's technique, all air contact is to be avoided and the harvesting syringe is rinsed with 0.5 ml of normal saline.

The calibre of the cannula should be 17 or 18G, atraumatic, and a 10 ml syringe should be used.

The favoured donor sites are the abdomen and lateral thighs (saddlebags).

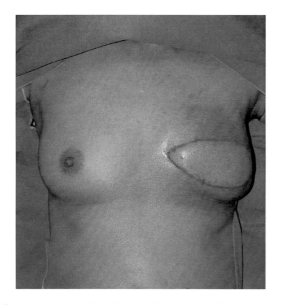

Fig. 7.1 Autologous latissimus dorsi flap with insufficient volume

A. Fitoussi et al., *Oncoplastic and Reconstructive Surgery for Breast Cancer*,
DOI: 10.1007/978-3-642-00144-4_7, © Springer-Verlag Berlin Heidelberg 2009

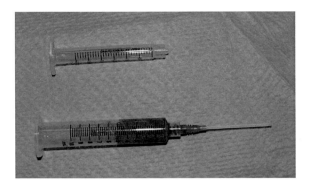

Fig. 7.2 Syringe for fat harvest

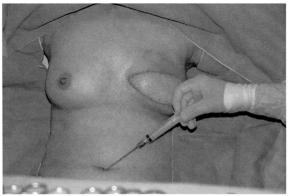

Fig. 7.3 Technique for fat harvesting

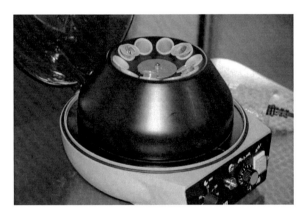

Fig. 7.4 Centrifugation

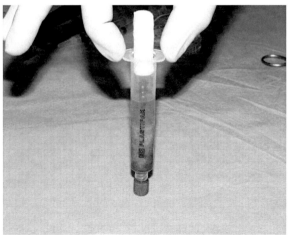

Fig. 7.5 The three layers following centrifugation

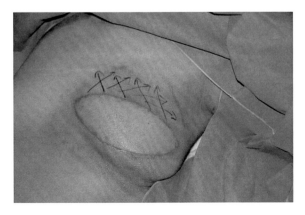

Fig. 7.6 Operative design

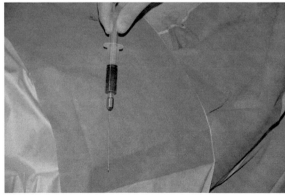

Fig. 7.7 Only the fat layer is retained for reinjection

Fat Preparation

The objective is to purify the fat, and at present centrifugation at 4,000 rpm for 3–4 min is recommended. This yields three different fractions. The lowest contains blood; the most superficial layer is oil; while the usable, purified adipocytes are found in the intermediate layer (Figs. 7.4 and 7.5).

Adipocyte Reinjection

Only the intermediate adipocyte-containing layer is transferred (Figs. 7.7–7.8).

Reinjection should be performed into the subcutaneous tissues and, ideally the muscle of a flap, due to its better vascularisation.

Several stab incisions are made into the breast skin to allow passage of the narrow-gauge (1.5 mm) cannulae.

The transfer of fat is made in multidirectional tunnels, from deep to superficial, according to the preoperative design (see Fig. 7.6). Microparticles of fat are thus injected into different planes in multiple and divergent directions in order to increase the surface contact area between the implanted cells and the recipient tissues, and thereby enhance the graft take.

The amount of fat transferred should be limited to avoid fat necrosis (Pierrefeu-Lagrange et al. 2006). It is therefore frequently necessary to repeat the procedure, and one should "overcorrect" (by about 140%) as a consequence of graft resorption. Although 30% is often quoted, our experience has shown that a greater loss—up to 40–60%—of the initial volume transferred is usual.

Whilst it is possible to transfer up to 450 cc of fat per breast, the most important element is homogeneous distribution of the fat in a three-dimensional "grid" to avoid poor graft take and subsequent steatonecrosis with contour deformity.

Postoperatively

Marked early swelling is common but this disappears within a couple of weeks.

Frequently, bruising is obvious in the zones of reinjection and lasts approximately three weeks.

One may judge the results at between three and six months after surgery; should a further procedure be required, it is usual to wait six months.

Discussion

Initially performed for the management of facial aging, indications for lipomodelage have spread into other areas of plastic surgery.

Two main indications of fat transfer can be described in breast surgery.

Volume Augmentation in the Autologous Flap-Reconstructed Breast

Transfer of purified adipocytes to the thoracomammary region for volume augmentation after autologous latissimus dorsi breast reconstruction was reported by Delay (2005) who coined the term "lipomodelage".

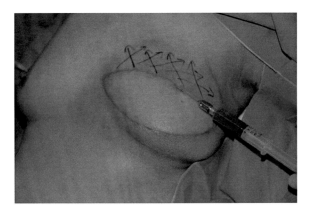

Fig. 7.8 Injection of fat cells

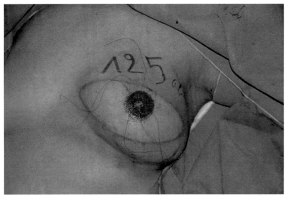

Fig. 7.9 Result with NAC reconstruction

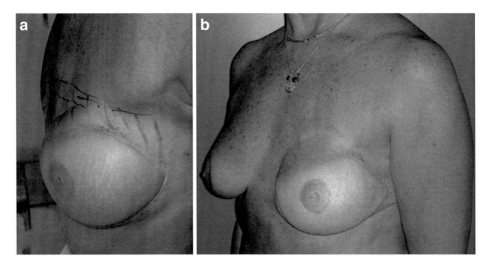

Fig. 7.10 a noticeable filling defect of the décolletage after latissimus dorsi breast reconstruction.
b much improved appearance following lipomodelage

Fat transfer represents a significant advance in autologous flap breast reconstruction for cancer: whether used for primary volume insufficiency or secondary atrophy in a latissimus dorsi flap, it may allow the avoidance of an implant in order to preserve a natural appearance and feel and, of course, the complications of a prosthesis. It is particularly good for filling defects of reconstructed breasts in the highly visible décolletage (Figures 7.10a and 7.10b). After good results were obtained in latissimus flaps, it was then extended to TRAM reconstructions.

In both cases, fat transfer is generally done during the second stage (i.e. nipple–areola reconstruction and contralateral symmetrisation).

Correction of Localised Deformities Following Either Implant-Based Reconstruction or Breast Conserving Therapy (ASBCT Grade 1)

In delayed implant breast reconstruction, some recommend pre-emptive fat transfer prior to reconstruction to improve the tissues and final aesthetic result (Delay et al. 2005; Spear et al. 2005). By the same token, fat transfer alone may be sufficient for small-volume breasts.

Treatment of secondary deformities including minor aesthetic sequelae of BCT (ASBCT Grade 1) raises questions about the scarring resulting from the reinjection of fat into the breast and a rigorous, high-quality surveillance.

In fact, since the 1980s, the use of autologous fat in breast surgery has been controversial, due to the development in the majority of some degree of cystosteatonecrosis and thus scarred areas and microcalcifications, rendering surveillance more difficult.

Microcalcifications and areas of cystosteatonecrosis are, however, typical after all breast surgery, and so radiological modifications are not unique to fat transfer. Frequently, imaging and an experienced radiologist are able to reliably differentiate between benign and suspect microcalcifications. MRI is useful for clarification in equivocal cases, but all solid lesions should be biopsied.

The technique of fat transfer must be rigorous and precise in order to reduce the risk of cystosteatonecrosis. The quantity of fat transferred and its distribution in the breast must be evaluated correctly.

Evaluation of fat transfer after conservative treatment of breast cancer remains in progress, and it's innocuousness must be demonstrated with respect to screening for recurrence.

Another controversial aspect of this technique concerns resorption of the fat: ever since autologous adipocytes were first used to correct volume, surgeons have reported variability in the results over time. At the end of the 1980s, it was appreciated that, in order to obtain a satisfactory result, injections should be small in volume but repeated.

Different techniques have been used to try and quantitatively evaluate the degree of fat resorption (photography, echography, CT and MRI). Overall, studies suggest resorption of around 50% of the initial volume in the first six months, followed by stabilisation.

Evolution of technical modifications, championed by Coleman, led to improved results. The principle aim of harvesting should be the least trauma possible. Purified fat should be reinjected in small aliquots so as to allow adipocytes to be in contact with vascularised tissue, avoiding large clumps that will not take. In any case, there will be a degree of fat resorption that the surgeon must anticipate and re-evaluate in the initial 3–6 months following the procedure.

Lipomodelage is ideal for improving the results of prosthetic reconstruction either postoperatively, injecting fat at the level of the frequently observed superior and superomedial décolletage defects, or during surgery in order to improve the quality of thoracic skin prior to secondary breast reconstruction by implant.

Complete Autologous Fat Transfer for Reconstruction of the Small Breast

When the native breast is of small volume, lipomodelage is ideal for autologous reconstruction. Whilst is requires several operative sittings, the patient may avoid the complications associated with prostheses and the donor site morbidity of musculocutaneous flaps (Fig. 7.11).

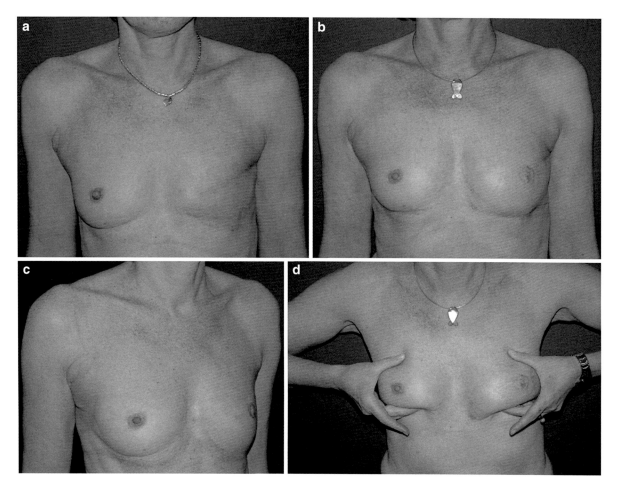

Fig. 7.11 **a** appearance of breast after first session of lipomodelage for delayed breast reconstruction. **b** breast following repeat lipomodelage and NAC reconstruction **c** breast following repeat lipomodelage and repeat areolar tattooing. **d** demonstration of the natural appearance and behaviour of the totally autogenous breast reconstruction

Conclusion

Fat transfer is a surgical technique and must be performed as such, respecting the fact that it is also a precise technique. It constitutes a real advance in the volumetric corrections that we can offer our breast reconstruction patients through autologous flaps or implants, and in the correction of aesthetic sequelae of breast conserving therapy of breast cancer. Its efficacy is no longer questioned by surgeons who practice this technique, but its safety remains to be evaluated.

References

Coleman SR, Saboeiro AP (2007) Fat grafting to the breast revisited: safety and efficacy. Plast Reconstr Surg 119(3):775–85; discussion: 786–7

Delay E, Delaporte T, Sinna R (2005) Alternative aux prothèses. Ann Chir Plast Esthet 50(5):652–72

Fournier PF (1985) Microlipoextraction et microlipoinjection. Rev Chir Esthet Lang Fr 10:40

Illouz YG (1986) The fat cell "graft": a new technique to fill depressions. Plast Reconstr Surg 78:122

Mojallal A, Foyatier JL (2004) Historique de l'utilisation du tissu adipeux comme produit de comblement en chirurgie plastique. Ann Chir Plast Esth 49:419–25

Pierrefeu-Lagrange AC, Delay E, Guerin N, Chekaroua K, Delaporte T (2006) Évaluation radiologique des seins reconstruits ayant bénéficié d'un lipomodelage. Ann Chir Plast Esthet 51:18–28

Sinna R, Delay E, Garson S, Mojallal A (2006) La greffe de tissu adipeux: mythe ou réalité scientifique. Lecture critique de la littérature. Ann Chir Plast Esth 51:223–30

Société Française de Chirurgie Plastique Reconstructrice et Esthétique (2004) Réinjection de graisse autologue ou lipofilling ou Lipostructure. Ann Chir Plast Esthet 49:456–8

Spear SL, Wilson HB, Lockwood MD (2005) Fat injection to correct contour deformities in the reconstructed breast. Plast Reconstr Surg 116(5):1300–5

Prophylactic Surgery

Today, genetics is part of the management of breast cancer, especially with families at risk. In fact, a growing number carry a genetic anomaly favouring breast cancer development (BRCA1 and 2), which increases the indications for prophylactic surgery.

Improved surveillance due, to six-monthly MRI scans, does not reduce the risk of cancer in these young women, but may reduce tumour size at diagnosis.

Recent data has shown a reduction of the order of 90–95% in the risk of developing cancer after prophylactic, or 'risk-reducing' surgery (Stefanek et al. 2001). Such information has led to a broadening of the indications for immediate breast reconstruction.

The complexity of breast cancer management has prompted the formation of multidisciplinary teams ("women at risk" groups comprising a geneticist, gynaecologist, psychologist and oncological and plastic surgeons) in order to best tailor therapeutic strategies to individual clinical situations.

The indications vary according to each particular case and individual and/or family history:

1. For mutated patients without cancer, a bilateral mastectomy with immediate implant-based reconstruction (should the patient wish) is the most frequent. Another reconstructive technique may sometimes be suggested according to the morphology of the patient. NAC preservation can also be offered if the patient desires, following discussion and informed consent for the slightly increased risk of local recurrence.
2. For those already diagnosed with early-stage tumours (<2 cm and node-negative), the same protocol applies. An early decision allows avoidance of adjuvant radiotherapy in the majority of cases and allows an initial bilateral treatment with immediate reconstruction in a single operation.
3. For patients with more advanced stages (>2 cm or node-positive) that will benefit from irradiation, mastectomy with axillary dissection but without immediate reconstruction is preferred. Delayed reconstruction with a musculocutaneous flap is preferred, and the nonaffected breast is generally managed as third-stage surgery.
4. Patients in whom mutation is discovered subsequent to treatment with tumourectomy and radiotherapy are managed in the same fashion. If implant reconstruction is possible, it may be performed bilaterally at the same operative sitting. If a musculocutaneous flap is required, mastectomy and a latissimus dorsi are offered for the irradiated breast. After a 4–6 month interval, the nonaffected breast can be reconstructed immediately following mastectomy. One may also suggest, depending on the morphology and personal preference of the patient, immediate bilateral TRAM flap reconstruction.
5. With an additional cancer of the contralateral breast, mastectomy with or without immediate reconstruction according to the same protocol may be considered.

The contralateral breast may be managed subsequently with a reconstruction adapted to the local conditions (usually a musculocutaneous flap because of local irradiation).

Reconstruction of the two NACs is best performed at another time, after volume reconstitution and stabilisation of the breast mounds.

Other less standardised situations arise and must be discussed within a group specialised in the management of mutated patients. These protocols are discussed fully with patients before the final decision is made.

The results of bilateral prophylactic surgery with different techniques are presented in Plate 8.1.

A. Fitoussi et al., *Oncoplastic and Reconstructive Surgery for Breast Cancer,*
DOI: 10.1007/978-3-642-00144-4_8, © Springer-Verlag Berlin Heidelberg 2009

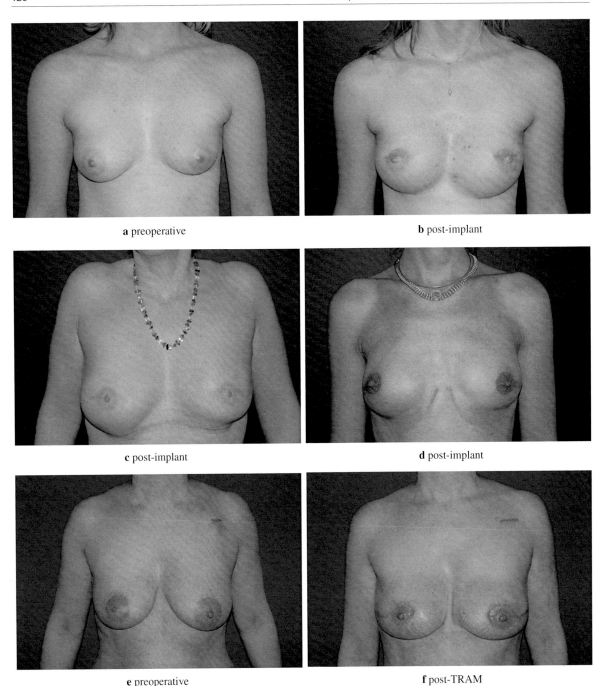

a preoperative   b post-implant

c post-implant   d post-implant

e preoperative   f post-TRAM

Plate 8.1 Results of bilateral prophylactic surgery

References

Stefanek M, Hartmann L, Nelson W (2001) Risk-reduction mastectomy: clinical issues and research needs. J Natl Cancer
   Inst 93:1297–1306

Radiotherapy After Breast Reconstruction

Introduction

Reconstructive surgical techniques are becoming more and more sophisticated, and breast cancer patients are becoming ever more demanding. Naturally, the choice of an immediate breast reconstruction must not compromise optimal locoregional and systemic treatment. When local treatment requires mastectomy and the patient requests immediate reconstruction (IBR), a preliminary multidisciplinary agreement is indispensable to evaluate the need for radiotherapy and its effects on the selected reconstruction.

Radiotherapy After Implant-Based Reconstruction

When radiotherapy is required for an implant-based breast reconstruction, the patient must be informed of the risk of alteration in the aesthetic result; particularly an increased risk of further surgery (Contant et al. 2000). It is difficult to evaluate aesthetic outcomes because the majority of studies report small patient populations, which are often heterogeneous with only a few patients per group (Contant et al. 2000; Chu et al. 1992). However, some experimental studies of prostheses themselves have demonstrated that a delivered dose of 50 Gy causes a loss of elasticity of the silicone gel (Klein and Kuske 1993). Contant et al. (2000) evaluated the toxicity of radiotherapy in 13 patients with implants in situ and 15 inserted after irradiation.

In 21% of cases, the authors observed cutaneous retraction and recommended autologous tissue techniques for cases requiring postoperative radiotherapy.

Faucher et al. (1998) reported 67 cases: 59 patients with an implant reconstruction after chest wall irradiation, and eight whose prosthesis was irradiated in situ. They did not show a significant alteration in the aesthetic appearance in the latter group, which unfortunately rapidly developed metastases that—with a mean survival of only six months—precluded long-term surveillance.

Another important issue is the definition of radiotherapy target volume after implant reconstruction. The target volume comprises the mastectomy scar, the gland-covering skin and the underlying pectoralis muscle, in addition to any gland remnants not removed during surgery. The thickness of the thoracic wall varies both within and between patients. In those with prostheses the volume is altered further, and in some a significant pulmonary and/or cardiac volume is unavoidably included in the radiation beam, which may create technical difficulties in trying to prevent long-term toxic effects (Kirova et al. 2007). In all cases, a dose tailored to each patient is essential (Fig. 9.1).

The junction of breast and nodal irradiation fields also poses technical problems with prostheses in situ when nodal irradiation is required (Kirova et al. 2006). One may see hot spots (where the dose is higher) on the dosing scan, which increase the incidence of late complications. It is important to respect international recommendations and quality-control criteria for irradiation in all cases (ICRU 1993, 1999; Fourquet et al. 2000). Despite these measures, Ringberg et al. (1999) have reported a 71% (10/14 patients) severe skin retraction rate. It is difficult to evaluate the results using self-completion satisfaction questionnaires, as

A. Fitoussi et al., *Oncoplastic and Reconstructive Surgery for Breast Cancer,*
DOI: 10.1007/978-3-642-00144-4_9, © Springer-Verlag Berlin Heidelberg 2009

Fig. 9.1 Field calculation for chest wall irradiation with in situ prosthesis

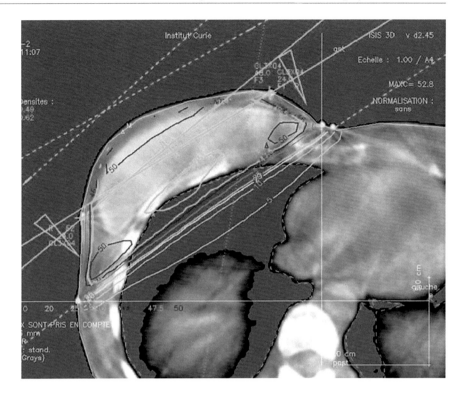

this same study stated that 85% of patients were satisfied with the aesthetic results for the reconstructed breast (Fourquet et al. 2000). A recent publication studied the problem in 114 patients after immediate implant-based reconstruction, with 44 of them having been irradiated and with a four-year follow up (Ringberg et al. 1999). The authors reported a threefold increase in the adverse capsular contraction rate in those irradiated (38.6%) compared to nonirradiated (14.1%), $p < 0.001$.

The Michigan Cancer Centre studied the rate of complications after retropectoral implant-based IBR with and without radiotherapy, in addition to patient satisfaction (Krueger et al. 2001). The population comprised 81 patients: 19 of which received radiotherapy to a total dose (including the mastectomy scar supplement) of 60.4 (50–66) Gy in 1.8–2 Gy fractions. With a median follow up of 31 months, complications were seen in 68% with and 31% without irradiation ($p = 0.006$). Radiotherapy was recognised as being a risk factor for failure of the reconstructive procedure ($p = 0.005$), as was tamoxifen ($p = 0.01$). It is worth noting that, in this study, radiotherapy did not appear to be a factor that predicted lack of patient satisfaction with their aesthetic outcome.

Radiotherapy after Musculocutaneous Flap Reconstruction

As a result of earlier studies, some authors suggest, that patients refusing mastectomy without IBR should be offered an autologous tissue reconstruction. In these cases, even with irradiation, the risk of complications is low. A study compared patients treated with conservative surgery to those with mastectomy and reconstruction (either immediate or delayed) with autologous tissue. They reported excellent rates of satisfaction in the mastectomy group (Dian et al. 2007). This study should be interpreted with care, however, as it only studied 70 patients.

Conclusion

When local treatment necessitates a mastectomy and the patient desires an immediate breast reconstruction, preliminary agreement by the multidisciplinary team is indispensable in order to evaluate the need for radiotherapy. When radiotherapy is required and the patient expresses a strong desire for IBR, the surgeon should favour the use of autologous tissue techniques, and the radiotherapist must adapt the techniques to the morphology of the patient.

Reconstruction and Medical Treatments

The aim of systemic adjuvant treatment in breast cancer is essentially to reduce the risk of metastasis, in addition to ensuring local control by surgery and radiotherapy. Systemic treatment will also have an impact upon preventing local recurrence (Punglia et al. 2007). Medical treatment interacts with oncoplastic surgery and reconstruction at different phases of the therapeutic pathway. The principal problem concerns the secondary effects of conventional cytotoxic chemotherapy. With immediate reconstruction, a prolonged postoperative recovery has the potential to delay adjuvant treatment. With delayed reconstruction, the procedure must be planned taking into account the schedule of systemic adjuvant treatment, and must therefore incorporate a safe interval in order to reduce the risk of complications: undue proximity to systemic therapy may cause postoperative difficulties. Finally, with neoadjuvant medical treatments, the aim is to reduce tumour volume, thereby allowing a conservative surgical treatment when a positive clinical response occurs.

Cytotoxic Chemotherapy

Adjuvant Treatment

The recommended duration of adjuvant chemotherapy is based on the most recent meta-analyses performed by the Oxford group (EBCTCG 2005): ideally from four to six months, and including if possible anthracyclines (Adriamycin and its derivatives). Addition of taxanes (Taxotere or paclitaxel, Taxol) shows a benefit in overall survival for patients with positive axillary nodes. The use of taxanes remains the subject of debate in node-negative patients (Colozza et al. 2006). In delayed reconstruction, and without adjuvant radiotherapy, we therefore recommend an interval from the latest chemotherapy—after recuperation from the

secondary haematological effects—of a minimum of four weeks. With irradiation following adjuvant chemotherapy, the interval is based primarily on the requirements of irradiation and its sequelae. Immediate reconstruction generated concerns about the risk of deferring adjuvant chemotherapy due to problems with postoperative healing (Taylor et al. 2005). For others, despite the increased risk of complications (between 15 and 27%), immediate breast reconstruction did not delay adjuvant therapy, as the complications generally arose in the first three postoperative weeks (Azuar 2007). It may be necessary to reintervene rapidly in cases of implant exposure/extrusion or partial flap necrosis (Azuar 2007).

Most studies report retrospective analyses of a limited number of patients from single centres. Chemotherapy does not seem to be associated with a significant increase in the rate of postoperative complications (Yule et al. 1996, Munhoz et al. 2005). These studies in general confirmed the absence of an adverse effect on recurrence-free and overall survival in immediate reconstruction, but statistical power was lacking. They also showed no significant increase in starting chemotherapy. In Mortenson's series, of 128 patients analysed in four subgroups (with or without immediate reconstruction; with or without adjuvant chemotherapy), the rate of postoperative complications was significantly increased after reconstruction compared to mastectomy alone ($p=0.02$), but chemotherapy was not delayed (Mortenson et al. 2004). Similarly, in the Milan group's series of 102 patients (Rey et al. 2005), the delay after immediate reconstruction was 54, compared to 60 days without reconstruction ($p=0.13$). The increase in infectious complications was related to the dose of chemotherapy rather than surgical interventions. In Allweis' series, chemotherapy was similarly delayed in patients not undergoing reconstruction: 53 vs. 41 days with reconstruction ($p=0.039$) (Allweis et al. 2002). The reason for this difference appears to be the younger age of those undergoing reconstruction (46 vs. 55 years; $p < 0.001$).

Taylor's study of 44 patients undergoing reconstruction followed by chemotherapy, compared to 49 controls, showed a mean increase in delay of only five days, due predominantly to healing problems (Taylor and Kumar 2005). A series of 95 patients published by Wilson et al. showed no delay in chemotherapy (Wilson et al. 2004). Finally, the Institut Gustave Roussy's series of 48 patients with IBR compared to 181 controls showed comparable delays (26 vs. 23 days; $p = 0.11$) (Gouy et al. 2005).

In the analysis of potential risk of delay for adjuvant chemotherapy, one must bear in mind that any adverse impact on survival remains controversial. In fact, only one study has shown a less favourable prognosis for recurrence-free survival when treatment is started more than 21 days after surgery. However, this was only found in the subgroup of nonmenopausal patients with hormone-receptor negative tumours (Colleoni et al. 2000); delayed chemotherapy was not significant in their other subgroups. Similarly, recent English, Spanish, Canadian and Danish retrospective studies were in agreement (Shannon et al. 2003; Jara Sanchez et al. 2007; Cold et al. 2005; Lohrisch et al. 2006), apart from when the intervals were greater than 12 weeks postoperatively (Lohrisch et al. 2006).

Neoadjuvant Chemotherapy

The only clinical benefit demonstrated with preoperative ("neoadjuvant") chemotherapy for inoperable tumours (excluding inflammatory and locally-advanced tumours) is an increase in breast conservation (Mauri et al. 2005; Kaufmann et al. 2006). No trial or meta-analysis has shown a significant difference in overall survival when the same treatment is given either as neoadjuvant or adjuvant (Jones and Smith 2006). The rates of conservation are increased when the tumour shows a clinical response, is less than 2 cm after chemotherapy, and is not lobular (Loibl et al. 2006). The rate of breast conservation is also increased with oncoplastic techniques (Clough et al. 2003) when the clinical response is inadequate or the tumour is located centrally. An increased risk of recurrence after neoadjuvant chemotherapy and conservative surgery has been reported, but tends to affect younger patients (under 35–40 years) (Oh et al. 2006) or those with radiotherapy alone and no surgery (Mauri et al. 2005; Ring et al. 2003). Routine mastectomy in these young patients, which yields a similar result is advocated by some (Kaufmann et al. 2006).

Immediate reconstruction after surgery following neoadjuvant chemotherapy is a recommended option, however, indications for postoperative irradiation should be determined by the initial tumour characteristics. In a series of 31 patients undergoing flap reconstruction after neoadjuvant chemotherapy, 17 (55%) experienced postoperative complications (Deutsch et al. 1999), however, this led to repeated postoperative chemotherapy in only two cases (6%). In a series of 1,195 flap reconstructions in 952 patients, some had received neoadjuvant chemotherapy. This was an independent predictor of complications, particularly healing problems and fat necrosis (Mehrara et al. 2006), but were considered to be minor.

Hormonotherapy

Adjuvant hormonotherapy is a standard treatment for patients with tumours that express hormone receptors (EBCTCG 2005). Options include aromatase inhibitors for postmenopausal patients and tamoxifen for premenopausal patients. Treatment duration is at least five, which is extended in certain cases to ten, years with tamoxifen subsequent (Colozza et al. 2006). The tolerance profile of these treatments with respect to neutropaenia or healing problems does not seem to interfere with surgical interventions. Preoperative hormonotherapy also allows an increased rate of breast conservation in those with a tumour that responds sufficiently well (Jones and Smith 2006). The use of tamoxifen may, however, have a deleterious effect on aesthetic outcome with concomitant irradiation (Deutsch and Flickinger 2003). The accrued risk of thrombosis with tamoxifen should be noted (Caine et al. 2003). With immobilisation due to surgery in combination with other risk factors, one must be more vigilant in those taking tamoxifen as either an adjuvant or a preventive measure.

Targeted Therapies

Trastuzumab (Herceptin)

Adjuvant immunotherapy with a monoclonal antibody targeting the oncogene *HER2* in patients overexpressing this receptor (approximately 20% of breast cancers: Romond et al. 2005; Smith et al. 2007) has recently been shown to produce a highly significant reduction in recurrence and mortality. The recommended duration of treatment (given intravenously every three weeks) is one year from the initial injection, given after the end of adjuvant or neoadjuvant chemotherapy. Trastuzumab is very well tolerated, aside from a limited risk of reduction in myocardial ejection fraction. There have been no reports of it interfering with reconstructive surgery, causing neither neutropaenia nor healing problems. A possible inductive effect of surgery on tumour cell HER2 proliferation has been suggested, giving a biological rationale to the supplementary use of this drug preoperatively (Tagliabue et al. 2003). Trastuzumab combined with neoadjuvant chemotherapy allows a considerable increase in the rate of complete clinical responses and potentially conservative treatment (Coudert et al. 2007; Buzdar et al. 2007).

Anti-angiogenetics

One of the most rapidly evolving medical oncological treatments involves agents targeting tumour neoangiogenesis, but there is the theoretical problem of interfering with reconstructive surgery using these products. Bevacizumab (Avastin), a monoclonal antibody targeting vascular endothelial growth factor (VEGF), obtained its marketing licence for breast cancer by demonstrating a survival benefit without progression of initial metastasis in association with weekly paclitaxel (Taxol) (Miller et al. 2007).

Several studies are in progress to investigate the use of bevacizumab as either an adjuvant or neoadjuvant therapy in breast cancer, but delayed healing, bleeding and thrombotic problems have been reported (Eskens and Verweij 2006). Because it has a half-life of about 20 days, and based on experiences in hepatic resection of colonic tumours, it is recommended that the drug should be stopped 6–8 weeks prior to major surgery. Potential postoperative complications in oncological and reconstructive surgery for breast cancer are not known and may be confirmed if the trials in progress validate anti-VEGF as an adjuvant treatment. Its optimal duration as an adjuvant treatment is yet to be determined. Testing of other drugs targeting VEGF signal transduction—including sorafenib (Nexavar) or sunitinib (Sutent)—in the metastatic phase has only recently begun.

In conclusion, immediate reconstructive surgery, even if it seems to increase postoperative complications, does not appear to be a major risk factor in delaying the start of adjuvant chemotherapy. Neoadjuvant treatments (chemo-, hormono- and immunotherapy) allow an increase in the rate of breast conservation without compromising overall survival, and may be complemented with oncoplastic techniques. If the new molecules acting on tumour neoangiogenesis are to be integrated as neoadjuvant or adjuvant therapies, specific evaluation of their impact on the postoperative period of reconstructive surgery will be required.

Psycho-oncological Aspects

Introduction

For patients facing it, breast surgery for cancer is often a difficult step in the course of their care. A radical surgical intervention such as mastectomy (without reconstruction) or repair (in the case of reconstruction) frequently has psychological repercussions.

Breast reconstruction has clearly progressed and there are now a wide variety of techniques available to the surgeon. However, perhaps in contrast to our own intuition, reconstruction does not remove the psychological sequelae. This treatment initially assails the woman with the loss of a particularly important part of her body, and then with its transformation. It is important to be aware that, sooner or later, these physical changes lead to significant psychological reorganisations aimed at ameliorating her fears and her satisfaction with the clinical management.

Psychological Experience of Cancer and Breast Surgery

Past History of Breast Cancer

Breast cancer, because of its real risk of death, raises the spectre of mortality, and such a diagnosis provokes diverse psychological reactions, often with an inability to assimilate medical information during consultations. The consequent emotional manifestations, which may be a concern in other circumstances, are "normal" defence reactions to the stress of a cancer diagnosis.

Full awareness of the illness and its effects does not develop immediately upon diagnosis. In fact, many women only really realise that they have cancer later; for some, this occurs only after mastectomy. Surgery assails them with both the possibility of mortality and the reality of losing a part of themselves.

Studies have evaluated the impact of breast cancer on the lives of those affected. One, involving a large sample of 817 with a 67% response rate, demonstrated completely satisfactory physical and emotional well-being 5–10 years after treatment, with only minor alterations (Ganz et al. 2002). The frequency of sexual activity diminished with time, and the use of adjuvant treatment (chemo- or hormonotherapy) was a predictive factor for reduced quality of life. An earlier study showed a better quality of life compared to patients with other chronic somatic problems, but an alteration of sexual function and conjugal relations between the first and second consecutive years after treatment, and a particular need for assistance with body image and reduced sexual interest issues (Ganz et al. 1996). A capacity to retain constructive and positive aspects of their experience of cancer contributes to a better quality of life. While most women rediscover a satisfactory level of well-being after cancer treatment, it nevertheless causes difficulties to some. Another study emphasised the negative impact, with respect to body image, of mastectomy with reconstruction compared to conservative treatment, as well as the particularly negative effects of chemotherapy on overall quality of life, particularly in young women (Janz et al. 2005).

Mastectomy

Mastectomy is a mutilating gesture that affects the body's integrity in its entirety and can impact on one's identity. For many women, mastectomy also symbolises an attack on the feminine and sexual identity (Lehmann 2007). They feel embarrassed by their physical appearance (naked or clothed), embarrassed compared to others; they feel that they have lost some of their sexual attractiveness or appeal, and can even develop feelings of being a "monster". Such emotions may be associated with relatively severe anxiety or depression (Kornblith and Ligibel 2003).

For some patients, difficulties in accepting the mutilation or loss of a particularly important body part can sometimes result in a state akin to mourning, similar to the loss of a loved one. Whilst this may be clinically obvious, its psychological impact is highly variable from one woman to another. In fact, for some women, the breast is a very important sexual organ that contributes significantly to both harmony and intimate life. For others, being a "woman" is a more general concept and is not necessarily so strongly defined by body image or sexual attributes. Also, reactions vary greatly between women, depending on personality, individual history and the type and quality of relationships formed with her partner and those close to her before the appearance of cancer. Alternatively, some women start to consider the breast a "bad" part when affected by cancer. It provides a constant reminder of the disease and may become the source of chronic anxious preoccupations if preserved. This causes certain patients to express an explicit desire for removal of the organ that is "responsible" and evokes a feeling of relief after the mastectomy because of its radical and secure appearance (Boussard et al. 2006).

Most studies comparing mastectomy to conservative surgery have not observed a major difference in overall quality of life (Schover 2004). In fact, whilst mastectomy can destroy the body image, emotional and physical problems seem to arise primarily from being faced with a potentially mortal illness. However, women undergoing mastectomy seem to experience more problems with physical functioning: muscle stiffness, sensitivity of the breast, pain, fatigue and concentration difficulties (Ganz et al. 2004). A recent large study (2,208 women) of breast cancer patients commencing radiotherapy indicated more problems with body image in the mastectomy group, but arm symptoms were more common following a tumourectomy (Hopwood et al. 2007). The type of surgery seems to have little impact on the overall quality of life.

Reconstruction

Breast reconstruction and the numerous technical advances seen today represent major progress in the surgical treatment of breast cancer. This allows us to respond to women's high expectations with respect to reconstruction. They are also known to assess repair of mutilation at both the aesthetic and psychological levels.

Overall, mastectomy with breast reconstruction is associated with better results in terms of psychosocial morbidity (anxiety, depression, body image, sexuality, self-esteem) and overall satisfaction than simple mastectomy. For this reason, it must be offered each time mastectomy is required and when conditions allow (Al-Ghazal et al. 2000).

Next comes the important task of integrating and elaborating the psychological aspects. Mastectomy–reconstruction represents a strong emotional experience with diverse fears of cancer, of the future, of the functional and aesthetic impact, and also the reactions of loved ones (Brédart and Petit 2005). In all cases, a real process of change occurs. The patient is faced with the thought of "never again", which requires giving up a previous self image and allowing the gradual creation of a new one.

Not all women accept reconstruction. A French study (Ananian et al. 2004) questioned 181 women with breast cancer before mastectomy and showed that four-fifths opted for reconstruction (immediate in 83%) against one-fifth who chose simple mastectomy. A more restricted Australian study (Reaby 1998) identified certain factors in favour of choosing reconstruction: most important was the desire to "feel whole", ahead of avoiding external prostheses, the ability to dress normally, and the rediscovery of femininity. The following factors were related to mastectomy alone: reconstruction was considered nonessential to physical or emotional well-being; information about reconstruction was not supplied; and reparative procedures were considered to be artificial.

Mastectomy with Immediate or Delayed Reconstruction

The processes in which immediate or delayed reconstruction are envisaged must be considered and ameliorated. A prospective, qualitative, multicentric English study analysed the style of decision-making when the choice between mastectomy and immediate or delayed reconstruction was made, and underlined the frequency of an instantaneous decision (without

time for reflection), which was primarily conditioned by the habitual surgical practice in that institution (Harcourt and Rumsey 2004). Following surgical intervention, psychological adaptation processes are not completed for a year, but despite the frequent shift in expectations occuring between the preoperative and postoperative periods, patients expressed a high level of satisfaction, focussing predominantly on the positive aspects of surgery. A retrospective study of 121 women who had chosen immediate over delayed reconstruction (Al-Ghazal et al. 2000) showed greater satisfaction in many aspects: anxiety, depression, body image, self-esteem. Another study (Elder et al. 2005) looked at reconstructed women and identified the avoidance of external prostheses as the principal factor. Roth's study (Roth et al. 2005) emphasised that those requesting immediate reconstruction presented an higher state of psychological distress than their delayed counterparts.

Similarly, with immediate reconstruction, some feel mutilated, with a reconstructed breast that is alien. Others felt that their female identity was under attack less intensely, and could more easily preserve their self-esteem. Other women complained of "everything moving too quickly", and regretted the lack of adequate time to reflect and understand the process. It may also be that the disillusionment involved in anticipating an unrealistic result (the breast being the same as before) is more important in the case of immediate reconstruction, where comparison is made with the breast's absence.

For delayed reconstruction, it is similarly important to inform patients of the existence of this possibility, even if not all choose it.

Prosthesis or Flap Techniques

When the surgeon has a range of various techniques, he/she presents those appropriate along with the advantages, disadvantages and risks of each. Many women resort to a prosthesis or expander, favouring the principle of less major surgery and a reduced peroperative risk. Others lean towards flap reconstruction, refusing to consider the use of exogenous material (potentially seen as a "foreign body"), and accepting in return the potential risks of a more major intervention.

The criteria for directing each patient should be explored in detail, as the surgeon relies on them to select the appropriate therapeutic option (Saulis et al. 2007).

Nipple Conservation

The psychological impact of this technique is currently poorly understood. The possibility of maintaining sensation in this area may positively affect sexuality, and it appears that women will be more satisfied with the intervention if they have been able to retain their nipples (Nahabedian and Tsangaris 2006).

After Reconstruction

Different aspects are taken into account to fully understand the role of breast reconstruction in the management of breast cancer (Bredart and Petit 2005).

Change and Its Consequences

Following reconstructive surgery, the woman's figure alters so habitual reference points will change. Some are afraid to look at themselves, to show their naked form, or even to touch the operated area. Some describe a loss of sensation in that part of their body: a loss of tactile sensation in the breast, as well as under the axilla in cases of dissection.

Functional Repercussions of Reconstruction

Many patients complain of intensely painful sensations secondary to mastectomy–reconstruction, in particular with flap-based reconstructions. These include a perception of pain, numbness or other disagreeable sensations (tension, pressure, contractions etc) leading to physical discomfort, in addition to the ever-present worry of disease recurrence that is triggered by such symptoms.

These painful sensations may last many months, despite effective analgesia. The processes that lead to chronic postoperative pain are complex and chronicity is correlated with their presence acutely. Therefore,

particular attention must be paid to them with referral to a postoperative pain specialist if required.

Aesthetic Consequences of Reconstruction

Reconstructive surgery is often associated with higher expectations regarding the aesthetic outcome than in those who undergo conservative surgery. Whilst cosmetic criteria are very important considerations, the surgeon must make the distinction between reconstructive, reparative and cosmetic surgery clear to each patient.

Impact of Reconstructive Surgery

Some studies have sought to evaluate the impact of reconstruction for breast cancer from different aspects including body image, self-esteem, identity and sexuality. In principle, reconstruction favours the adaptive processes that permit psychological acceptance.

Quality of Life Studies

Quality of life studies show that for the majority of women breast reconstruction improves the quality of life compared to simple mastectomy (but is lower than for conservative treatment). The most significant differences affect the physical aspect of body image as well as the psychological aspect of self-esteem. Ultimately this impacts on the overall quality of life, thus certain aspects may remain altered over the long term (Ganz 2002, 2004) (Kraus 1999). The study performed by Elder et al. (2005) found that quality of life at one year was comparable to that of the general population.

Another study of 1957 patients questioned 1–5 years after cancer showed that reconstruction was more common in younger women, those with a higher level of education, and those with a partner. Mastectomy and reconstruction were found to be comparable with respect to physical symptoms and quality of life, but negative sexual consequences were more frequent in reconstruction (Rowland et al. 2000). However, it suggested that the age of the patient (younger) and the type of adjuvant treatment (chemotherapy) are influential factors in this difference, rather than simply the reconstruction itself. In young women in particular, mastectomy with or without reconstruction is more often associated with body image issues (Fobair et al. 2006).

Satisfaction with Reconstructive Surgery

Overall satisfaction with reconstructive surgery underlines the importance of acknowledging any preoperative psychological distress and somatic preoccupation as these can negatively influence the overall and aesthetic satisfaction postoperatively (Roth et al. 2007). This evaluation should also be performed at different postoperative times because satisfaction evolves with time and the temporal sequence is not well understood (Alderman et al. 2000).

Overall, the literature shows that satisfaction with conservative surgery is always higher than with mastectomy, whether reconstruction has been performed or not (Rowland et al. 2000). An evaluation of satisfaction with regard to different reconstructive techniques (Alderman et al. 2000, 2007; Wilkins et al. 2000) in the Michigan Breast Reconstruction Outcomes Study (212 patients. 1994 and 1997) revealed a reduction in general satisfaction over time, but the continued superiority of aesthetic satisfaction in women with flap reconstruction compared to prostheses or expanders.

Prophylactic Surgery in Women at Genetic Risk

These are very particular situations involving women from high-risk families, either with or without the identification of a genetic mutation. These women have either already been diagnosed with a breast or ovarian cancer or not, but the familial genetic predisposition leaves them at high risk. They are often marked by a strong family history of cancers, and deaths therefrom, thus their outlook is particularly pessimistic. Such women often seek any way to try and escape their family history and survive cancer, and are determined to explore the notion of prophylactic surgery.

They are often well-informed and demanding and may run up against a lack of understanding from others, notably those unaware of their family context or lacking knowledge of genetic risk. If this lack of understanding emanates from the medical body, the burden is even heavier to bear.

More than ever in this context, one must understand the woman's values and preferences (Charles et al. 1997), and provide her with a means for communicating with the clinicians that facilitates fully informed consent. One should not diminish the patient's concerns regarding the impact of any decision on partners and other family members. Do not forget also that the information considered by the patient during her treatment is also of great value to those potentially impacted by the same genetic risk. The patient serves as the "model" by example, and may be the initiator (direct or indirect) for requests for prophylactic surgery from others in the family.

The 2004 Cochrane report (Lostumbo et al. 2004) studying this question highlighted the lack of validated prospective studies in this area and reiterated the need for information. As to psychosocial impact, the report concluded there to be an overall satisfaction with respect to prophylactic surgery and a reduction in anxiety (in comparison with women who opt for surveillance) (Bresser et al. 2006). It identified, however, an adverse effect on body image, femininity and aesthetic satisfaction. Saulis' retrospective study (Saulis et al. 2007) demonstrated satisfaction in two-thirds of women three years after intervention, but persistent sexual consequences. It also underlined the paucity of long-term data. Lodder et al. (2002) concluded that the greater satisfaction was primarily attributable to the relief of risk reduction due to the intervention. Hopwood, in 2000, following a detailed evaluation of mental health and body image in risk-reduction mastectomy for breast cancer risk reduction, nevertheless underlined the importance of preparation prior to intervention and the need for long-term psychological follow up. In fact, while the majority of these women did not present notable psychological problems, more than half manifested difficulties arising from the alteration of body image, particularly when they experienced surgical complications.

According to Metcalfe et al. (2004a), the improved satisfaction and overall functioning in these women is, however, negatively affected by younger age, the presence of a strong family history and delayed reconstruction. Another study by the same author (Metcalfe et al. 2004b) correlated lower satisfaction with reconstruction to an overestimation of preoperative risk, so such patients should be assisted in effectively evaluating their personal risk in order to improve overall satisfaction with breast surgery.

Socio-emotional Environment of the Patient

Although the experience of cancer and breast surgery primarily affects the woman concerned, it is not without repercussions on her immediate surroundings: the partner, if she has one, and her family in general. It is very important to evaluate the functioning of the relationship of the couple prior to the cancer, any anxiety about the partner's attitude between diagnosis and deciding to undergo surgery and finally the manner of her participation in the choice of treatment (Reaby 1998). The manner in which the family communicates must also be taken into account, since it allows anticipation of the kind of environmental resources from which the patient might draw (Neill et al. 1998). In general, an isolated personality is widely recognised as a risk factor for psychological decompensation in women with cancer.

Apart from some qualitative experimental studies, often undertaken by nurses, the current literature is lacking in this regard and would benefit from being developed.

Practical Clinical Recommendations

Through their experience, and in collaboration with the clinical care teams, surgeons have developed a certain expertise in the arena of reconstructive breast surgery.

Detailed and personalised patient evaluation is fundamental because it allows any difficulties, and their negative psychological consequences, to be predicted and a rapid and appropriate response to be made. It is important to modulate the psychological responses and satisfaction of patients with regard to reconstruction (Roth et al. 2007).

This assessment always has its place in the process, developing according to the needs and expectations of each patient, and according to the specifics of different stages of treatment.

Certain tools are available for evaluation, presently primarily in a clinical research setting. The carers can easily find supporting information in their field of clinical practice, allowing them to prepare the consultation efficiently and be thorough without wasting time.

There are several evaluation tools:

– General: quality of life (EORTC QLQ-C30; Aaronson 1993) associated with the specific QLQ BR23 module for breast cancer, or care received (EORTC IN-PATSAT32)
– More specific in a particular dimension: depression (Zang's self-completion depression ladder; Dugan et al. 1998), body image scale (Brédart et al. 2007), self-esteem, sexuality or communication between the couple or the family

A number of recommendations may be extracted from the literature, and these concur with our experiences at the Institut Curie.

Prior to Surgery

The recommendations are as follows:

– Remember the importance of collaboration between the referring doctor and the hospital team in the framework of well-established preliminary care.
– A shared decision-making model is preferable, particularly when many surgical options are available (Ananian et al. 2004; Charles et al. 1997). Some qualitative evaluation has been preformed (Ganz et al. 1996; Neill et al. 1998).

In the context of breast reconstruction, the principle of "paternalistic" medicine (in other words, determining what is good for another person) can result in decisions with potentially serious consequences for the patient. For example, if the surgical intervention is selected solely by her surgeon, the patient may place full responsibility for the outcome on him, especially if she is frustrated and dissatisfied with it. Some studies have established a correlation between the feeling of being inadequately informed and the level of dissatisfaction (Saulis et al. 2007).

The shared-decision model is based on a partnership with exchange of information between clinician and patient: an in-depth exploration of values, preferences and expectations, and individualised information that allows a clear choice. For example, deciding that conservative treatment may be preferable just because of breast preservation and equivalent survival results may not necessarily reflect the preferences of all patients (Sepucha et al. 2007).

Communication between doctor and patient passes through different stages. Verbal information is personalised and individualised. This is complemented by written supporting information (Wolf 2004). The use of cancer plans has emphasised the information needs of cancer sufferers, and much effort has been expended in this regard. We use information leaflets at the Institut Curie, which have been refined according to a multidisciplinary model. These are given to the patient at the end of the consultation and in no way replace verbal information, rather complete and reinforce it. They also represent a written record to which the patient may return at a later time, either alone or with her partner.

Additional information may be provided in the form of photographs of previous procedures: this information should be presented on request. When the surgeon has such images, it is important to emphasise that they only represent examples, and stress the great variability of aesthetic results that occur from one woman to another, as there are many individual factors.

Some patients also wish to meet with women who have had such procedures previously. This should be encouraged for various reasons:

–	To confirm the validity of information. Although it is well-established scientifically that breast reconstruction leads to neither risk of recurrence nor its masking, some women remain concerned (Brédart and Petit 2005).
–	To aid with overall understanding of the benefits (for example, improved satisfaction with respect to body image), limitations (for example, a breast not being identical to that prior to surgery, and aesthetic results that are not perfect) and risks (surgical complications, requirement for revisional surgery) of breast reconstruction, in addition to what is expected of the patient herself. When therapeutic alternatives exist, it can also help with the patient's understanding of

immediate or delayed reconstruction and the surgery envisaged (Reaby 1998).
–	To help the patient prepare for the consequences of her decision, and more generally assist in conceptualising the surgery and its consequences.
–	To allow the patient sufficient time for reflection. In case of hesitation, meetings with others are offered, as is a second surgical opinion if required. This is particularly important in prophylactic surgery (Lalloo et al. 2000).
–	To evaluate the psychosocial context and degree of family support, notably from the partner. Ideally, the partner should be present during consultations at least once in order to meet and question the surgeon. Integration of the partner into surgical consultations reduces the risk of psychological difficulties and alterations in the sexual relationship between the couple (Morris 1980).
–	To confirm the absence of major psychological pathology; if necessary, a referral should be made to a psychologist for preliminary interview (Roth et al. 2007).

During Hospitalisation

The surgeon's visit represents an essential stage that allows clarification of the intervention and any final queries.

Other sources of support are now available, including accompaniment by the breast nurse (Boussard et al. 2006), and a consultation with the preoperative nurse (as is standard at the Institut Curie), who routinely welcomes the patients the night before their operation. Here, a lengthy individual interview is performed by one of the specialised nurses. The objectives of the interview are as follows:

–	To inform the patient of the available procedures and the course of their hospitalisation
–	To re-evaluate the patient's knowledge of her illness and the planned procedure
–	To help the patient re-express any questions
–	To address the patient's and/or family's anxieties
–	To direct the patient, according to her needs, towards the different members of the care team including the doctor, social worker, dietician, onco-psychologist (a psychologist or psychiatrist experienced in cancer) and so forth.

- To address the consequences of surgery on the patient's daily life, body image and femininity, and on the rapport between the couple
- To anticipate the return home

Postoperatively

The nurses assist the patient in progressively exposing the scar. Revealing the reconstruction represents an essential step in the integration of the new breast, and depends heavily on the experience of the nurses. Some patients are very apprehensive and not always aware of the local changes that will evolve in time post-operatively. Here, information provided by the surgeon and repeated by the carers is vitally important.

For those that need more time before being able to face the results of their surgery, it is preferable with the nurse, before discharge rather than finding themselves dealing with the situation alone at home.

Sometimes meeting with other patients may represent a source of moral support and useful guidance. Some, on the other hand, tend to withdraw into themselves and avoid this type of confrontation that they perceive as unduly frightening.

Onco-psychological Review

At this stage, the individual mechanisms of psychological adjustment must be carefully observed. They depend on numerous factors: representation of cancer, personality, general mode of adaptation, previous experience(s), stressful life events, and emotional and socioenvironmental support.

Preoperative intervention by the onco-psychologist is not always required. Many women present visible emotional reactions, which are culturally influenced. For others the required management may be satisfactorily delivered upon request, particularly at an early stage.

Certain situations involving psychological vulnerability, however, require psychological intervention at the time of hospitalisation, either at the request of the patient herself or the care team. These may include:

- The presence of a behavioural disorder that hinders management, a known psychological illness or, occasionally, the presence of suicidal ideation or behaviour.

- Patients querying the partner's acceptance of the procedure. This request often signifies a difficulty that the patient herself has with respect to the surgery, which needs to be worked on early, before envisaging later work with the couple.
- Patients raising questions about communicating with their children about the disease. Here, the patient herself may envisage a problem, or it may be identified by the care team.

For the special case of women undergoing prophylactic surgery due to genetic risk, most benefit from at least one preliminary meeting with the onco-psychologist (and others in the multidisciplinary team). Here, the interview often proves crucial to understanding the patient's decision and verifying her ability to anticipate the consequences—not only for herself, but also for her loved ones (Lalloo et al. 2000).

Affiliated Groups and Associations

A number of associations offer their services during hospitalisation, providing solid support, the exchange of experiences, and interviews with a network of other patients who have had similar experiences.

Postoperatively and Beyond

The surgeon and general practitioner should be in effective contact, in order to assure the continuity and uniformity of management both pre- and post-operatively.

One should not be afraid to warn the patient of the possibility of a period of psychological instability after the intervention; this equally in more favourable cases where the patient feels well-prepared. One can legitimise the psychological reactions that occur and confirm that they signal adaptive processes, especially in regard to intimate life.

Consultation with a psychologist or psychiatrist—ideally an onco-psychologist accustomed with breast cancer patients—should be offered to the patient. In most cases, one or two consultations suffice to assist with the integration of experiences and rehabilitation. They can initiate the processes of change, aiding the patient in relation to her altered identity, the impact of the intervention on the intimacy of the couple, and in establishing new reference points. They will allow the patient to better communicate with her close ones, because she is often in search of a better balance between the needs of her feelings and the desire to protect her family.

On the other hand, some patients find themselves in great psychological distress at the end of the process, and may require a more supportive psychological follow up. This is often the case with women who have had previous traumatic experiences (in more severe cases, it is not uncommon to find evidence of physical and/or psychological violence or physical or sexual abuse), or with women that suffer from significant socioemotional isolation.

In cases of significant perturbations in the intimate life of the couple, a consultation with a sexologist experienced with cancer patients may be offered. This knowledge of the potential sexual impact of cancer and its treatment is attracting growing interest from institutions, and some now suggest specialised consultations as a routine part of treatment. At the Institut Curie, a recent project showed that a multidisciplinary consultation comprising sexologist, gynaeco-endocrinologist and onco-psychologist in collaboration with the referring clinician assists in evaluating and managing difficulties encountered in the couple's intimate and sexual life.

For some years now, France and other countries have seen a strong growth in groups at the centre of oncology, which welcome patients, listen, and offer advice and orientation, as well as individual support or group meetings that are often enlivened by former patients. These days, more modern approaches to this issue involving the Internet—with its chat forums and blogs—are employed and have been adjudged both satisfactory and supportive by those that use them. They represent a useful source of information and support, and play an important psychological role in removing the stigma or marginalisation perceived in relation to cancer.

Conclusion

Breast reconstruction for cancer represents a complex, significant and perhaps lasting stage in the lives of those affected, as does their satisfaction with the treatments received. This can lead to significant and diverse psycho-affective effects on both the patient and her family, touching on body image, identity, sexuality and conjugal relations. This is why recommendations for good clinical practice increasingly include a multidisciplinary approach, an overall evaluation of the physical and psychological state of the patient preoperatively, a verification of her understanding of the surgical options available, and a communication strategy with her doctor that allows participation in decisions with as much autonomy as is possible. Certain precautions are required: allocating time to inform the patient and welcome her questions; leaving sufficient time for her decisions to mature; and, in all cases, necessitates psychological support undertaken by the doctor and referring team, or in more difficult cases by oncopsychologists that are used to dealing with these specific problems.

References

Aaronson NK, Ahmedzai S, Bergman B, et al. (1993) The European Organization for Research and Treatment of Cancer QLQ-C30: a quality-of-life instrument for use in international clinical trials in oncology. J Natl Cancer Inst 85:365–76

Al-Ghazal SK, Fallowfield L, Blamey RW (2000) Comparison of psychological aspects and patient satisfaction following breast conserving surgery, simple mastectomy and breast reconstruction. Eur J Cancer 36:1938–43

Al-Ghazal SK, Sully L, Fallowfield L, et al. (2000) The psychological impact of immediate rather than delayed breast reconstruction. Eur J Surg Oncol 26:17–9

Allweis TM, Boisvert ME, Otero SE, et al. (2002) Immediate reconstruction after mastectomy for breast cancer does not prolong the time to starting adjuvant chemotherapy. Am J Surg 183:218–21

Alderman AK, Wilkins EG, Lowery JC, et al. (2000) Determinants of patient satisfaction in postmastectomy breast reconstruction. Plast Reconstr Surg 106:769–76

Alderman AK, Kuhn LE, Lowery JC, et al. (2007) Does patient satisfaction with breast reconstruction change over time? Two-year results of the Michigan Breast Reconstruction Outcomes Study. J Am Coll Surg 204:7–12

Ananian P, Houvenaeghel G, Protière C, et al. (2004) Determinants of patients' choice of reconstruction with mastectomy for primary breast cancer. Ann Surg Oncol 11:762–71

Azuar P (2007) Oncoplastic surgery in breast cancer indications and results. Presse Med 36:341–456

Brédart A, Petit JY (2005) Partial mastectomy: a balance between oncology and aesthetics. Lancet Oncol 6:130

Brédart A, Razavi D, Robertson C, et al. (2001) A comprehensive assessment of satisfaction with care: internal consistency and validity testing across oncology settings from France, Italy, Poland and Sweden. Pat Educ Counsel 43:243–52

Brédart A, Verdier S, Waine A, Dolbeault S (2007) Traduction/adaptation Française de l'échelle "Body Image Scale" (BIS) évaluant la perception de l'image du corps chez des femmes atteintes de cancer du sein. Psycho-oncologie 1:24–30

Bresser PJ, Seynaeve C, Van Gool AR, et al. (2006) Satisfaction with prophylactic mastectomy and breast reconstruction in genetically predisposed women. Plast Reconstr Surg 117:1675–882

Boussard V, Capuano A, Borde-Müller G (2006) Les difficultés psychologiques liées à la chirurgie mammaire. Référentiels de l'Institut Curie

Buzdar AU, Valero V, Ibrahim NK, et al. (2007) Neoadjuvant therapy with paclitaxel followed by 5-fluorouracil, epirubicin, and cyclophosphamide chemotherapy and concurrent trastuzumab in human epidermal growth factor receptor 2-positive operable breast cancer: an update of the initial randomized study population and data of additional patients treated with the same regimen. Clin Cancer Res 13:228–33

Caine GJ, Stonelake PS, Rea D (2003) Coagulopathic complications in breast cancer. Cancer 98:1578–86

Charles C, Gafni A, Whelan T (1997) Shared decision-making in the medical encounter: what does it mean? (or it takes at least two to tango). Soc Sci Med 44:681–92

Chu FCH, Kaufmann TP, Dawson GA, et al. (1992) Radiation therapy of cancer in prosthetically augmented or reconstructed breasts. Radiology 185:429–33

Cold S, During M, Ewertz M, et al. (2005) Does timing of adjuvant chemotherapy influence the prognosis after early breast cancer? Results of the Danish Breast Cancer Cooperative Group (DBCG). Br J Cancer 93:627–32

Colleoni M, Bonetti M, Coates AS, et al. (2000) Early start of adjuvant chemotherapy may improve treatment outcome for premenopausal breast cancer patients with tumors not expressing estrogen receptors. The International Breast Cancer Study Group. J Clin Oncol 18:584–90

Colozza M, de Azambuja E, Cardoso F, et al. (2006) Breast cancer: achievements in adjuvant systemic therapies in the pre-genomic era. Oncologist 11:111–25

Contant CM, van Geel AN, van der Holt B, et al. (2000) Morbidity of immediate breast reconstruction after mastectomy by subpectorally placed silicone prosthesis: the adverse effect of radiotherapy. Eur J Surg Oncol 26:344–50

Coudert BP, Largillier R, Arnould L, et al. (2007) Multicenter phase II trial of neoadjuvant therapy with trastuzumab, docetaxel, and carboplatin for human epidermal growth factor receptor-2-overexpressing stage II or III breast cancer: results of the GETN(A)-1 trial. J Clin Oncol 25:2678–84

Clough KB, Lewis JS, Couturaud B, et al. (2003) Oncoplastic techniques allow extensive resections for breast-conserving therapy of breast carcinomas. Ann Surg 237:26–34

Deutsch M, Flickinger JC (2003) Patient characteristics and treatment factors affecting cosmesis following lumpectomy and breast irradiation. Am J Clin Oncol 26:350–3

Deutsch MF, Smith M, Wang B, et al. (1999) Immediate breast reconstruction with the TRAM flap after neoadjuvant therapy. Ann Plast Surg 42:240–4

Dian D, Schwenn K, Mylonas I, et al. (2007) Aesthetic result among breast cancer patients undergoing autologous breast reconstruction versus breast conserving therapy. Arch Gynecol Obstet 275:445–50

Dugan W, Mac Donald M, Passik SD, et al. (1998) Use of the Zung self-rating depression scale in cancer patients: feasibility as a screening tool. Psycho-oncology 7:483–93

Early Breast Cancer Trialists' Collaborative Group (2005) Effects of chemotherapy and hormonal therapy for early breast cancer on recurrence and 15-year survival: an overview of the randomised trials. Lancet 365:1687–717

Elder EE, Brandberg Y, Björklund T, et al. (2005) Quality of life and patient satisfaction in breast cancer patients after immediate breast reconstruction: a prospective study. Breast 14:201–8

Eskens FA, Verweij J (2006) The clinical toxicity profile of vascular endothelial growth factor (VEGF) and vascular endothelial growth factor receptor (VEGFR) targeting angiogenesis inhibitors; a review. Eur J Cancer 42:3127–39

Faucher A, Dihuydy JM, Etcheberry TG, et al. (1998) Reconstruction mammaire prothétique et radiothérapie: analyse de 67 cas. Bull Cancer 85:167–72

Fobair P, Stewart SL, Chang S, et al. (2006) Body image and sexual problems in young women with breast cancer. Psycho-oncology 15:579–94

Fourquet A, Rosenwald JC, Campana F, et al. (2000) Radiotherapy of cancer of the breast. Technical problems and new approaches. Cancer Radiother Suppl 1:180s–186s

Ganz PA, Coscarelli A, Fred C, et al. (1996) Breast cancer survivors: psychosocial concerns and quality of life. Breast Cancer Res Treat 38:183–99

Ganz PA, Desmond KA, Leedham B, et al. (2002) Quality of life in long-term, disease-free survivors of breast cancer: a follow-up study. J Natl Cancer Inst 94:39–49

Ganz PA, Kwan L, Stanton AL, et al. (2004) Quality of life at the end of primary treatment of breast cancer: first results from the moving beyond cancer randomized trial. J Natl Cancer Inst 96:376–87

Gouy S, Rouzier R, Missana MC, et al. (2005) Immediate reconstruction after neoadjuvant chemotherapy: effect on adjuvant treatment starting and survival. Ann Surg Oncol 12:161–6

Harcourt D, Rumsey N (2004) Mastectomy patients' decision-making for or against immediate breast reconstruction. Psycho-oncology 13:106–15

Hopwood P, Lee A, Shenton A, et al. (2000) Clinical follow-up after bilateral risk reducing ("prophylactic") mastectomy: mental health and body image outcomes. Psycho-oncology 9:462–72

Hopwood P, Haviland J, Mills J, et al. (2007) The impact of age and clinical factors on quality of life in early breast cancer: an analysis of 2208 women recruited to the UK START Trial (Standardisation of Breast Radiotherapy Trial). Breast 16:241–51

ICRU (1993) Prescribing, recording, and reporting photon beam therapy (Report 50). International Commission on Radiation Units and Measurements, Washington, DC

ICRU (1999) Prescribing, recording, and reporting photon beam therapy (Report 62; supplement to Report 50). International Commission on Radiation Units and Measurements, Bethesda, MD

Janz NK, Mujahid M, Lantz PM, et al. (2005) Population-based study of the relationship of treatment and sociodemographics on quality of life for early stage breast cancer. Qual Life Res 14:1467–79

Jara Sanchez C, Ruiz A, Martin M, et al. (2007) Influence of timing of initiation of adjuvant chemotherapy over survival in breast cancer: a negative outcome study by the Spanish Breast Cancer Research Group (GEICAM). Breast Cancer Res Treat 101:215–23

Jones RL, Smith IE (2006) Neoadjuvant treatment for early-stage breast cancer: opportunities to assess tumour response. Lancet Oncol 7:869–74

Kaufmann M, Hortobagyi GN, Goldhirsch A, et al. (2006) Recommendations from an international expert panel on the use of neoadjuvant (primary) systemic treatment of operable breast cancer: an update. J Clin Oncol 24:1940–9

Kirova Y, Campana F, Fournier-Bidoz N, et al. (2007) Radiothérapie pour qui et comment? In: Morère JF (ed) Cancer du sein. Masson, Paris

Kirova YM, Servois V, Campana F, et al. (2006) CT-scan based localization of the internal mammary chain and supra clavicular nodes for breast cancer radiation therapy planning. Radiother Oncol 79:310–5

Klein EE, Kuske RR (1993) Changes in photon dose distribution due to breast prostheses. Int J Radiat Oncol Biol Phys 25:541–9

Kornblith A, Ligibel J (2003) Psychosocial and sexual functioning of survivors of breast cancer. Semin Oncol 30:799–813

Kraus PL (1999) Body image, decision making, and breast cancer treatment. Cancer Nurs 22:421–7

Krueger EA, Wilkins EG, Strawderman M, et al. (2001) Complications and patients satisfaction following expander/implant breast reconstruction with and without radiotherapy. Int J Radiat Oncol Biol Phys 49:713–21

Lalloo F, Baildam A, Brain A, et al. (2000) A protocol for preventative mastectomy in women with an increased lifetime risk of breast cancer. Eur J Surg Oncol 26:711–3

Lehmann A (2007) Incidences psychologiques de la chirurgie du sein. In: JY Petit, et al. Le cancer du sein, chirurgie diagnostique, curative et reconstructrice, updated 2nd edn. Arnette, Paris

Lodder LN, Frets PG, Trijsburg RW, et al. (2002) One year follow-up of women opting for presymptomatic testing for BRCA1 and BRCA2: emotional impact of the test outcome and decisions on risk management (surveillance or prophylactic surgery). Breast Cancer Res Treat 73:97–112

Lohrisch C, Paltiel C, Gelmon K, et al. (2006) Impact on survival of time from definitive surgery to initiation of adjuvant chemotherapy for early-stage breast cancer. J Clin Oncol 24:4888–94

Loibl S, von Minckwitz G, Raab G, et al. (2006) Surgical procedures after neoadjuvant chemotherapy in operable breast cancer: results of the GEPARDUO trial. Ann Surg Oncol 13:1434–42

Lostumbo L, Carbine N, Wallace J, et al. (2004) Prophylactic mastectomy for the prevention of breast cancer. Cochrane Database Syst Rev 4:CD002748

Mauri D, Pavlidis N, Ioannidis JP (2005) Neoadjuvant versus adjuvant systemic treatment in breast cancer: a meta-analysis. J Natl Cancer Inst 97:188–94

Mehrara BJ, Santoro TD, Arcilla E, et al. (2006) Complications after microvascular breast reconstruction: experience with 1195 flaps. Plast Reconstr Surg 118:1100–9; discussion 1110–1

Metcalfe KA, Esplen MJ, Goel V, et al. (2004a) Psychosocial functioning in women who have undergone bilateral prophylactic mastectomy. Psycho-oncology 13:14–25

Metcalfe KA, Semple JL, Narod SA (2004b) Satisfaction with breast reconstruction in women with bilateral prophylactic mastectomy: a descriptive study. Plast Reconstr Surg 114:360–6

Miller KD, Sledge GW, Burstein HJ (2007) Angiogenesis inhibition in the treatment of breast cancer: a review of studies presented at the 2006 San Antonio Breast Cancer Symposium. Clin Adv Hematol Oncol 5:1–12

Morris T (1980) Postoperative adjustment of patients with breast cancer. J R Soc Med 73:215–7

Mortenson MM, Schneider PD, Khatri VP, et al. (2004) Immediate breast reconstruction after mastectomy increases wound complications: however, initiation of adjuvant chemotherapy is not delayed. Arch Surg 139:988–91

Munhoz AM, Montag E, Fels KW, et al. (2005) Outcome analysis of breast-conservation surgery and immediate latissimus dorsi flap reconstruction in patients with T1 to T2 breast cancer. Plast Reconstr Surg 116:741–52

Neill KM, Armstrong N, Burnett CB (1998) Choosing reconstruction after mastectomy: a qualitative analysis. Oncol Nurs Forum 25:743–50

Nahabedian MY, Tsangaris TN (2006) Breast reconstruction following subcutaneous mastectomy for cancer: a critical appraisal of the nipple–areola complex. Plast Reconstr Surg 117:1083–90

Oh JL, Bonnen M, Outlaw ED, et al. (2006) The impact of young age on locoregional recurrence after doxorubicin-based breast conservation therapy in patients 40 years old or younger: how young is "young"? Int J Radiat Oncol Biol Phys 65:1345–52

Punglia RS, Morrow M, Winer EP, et al. (2007) Local therapy and survival in breast cancer. N Engl J Med 356:2399–405

Reaby LL (1998) Breast restoration decision making: enhancing the process. Cancer Nurs 21:196–204

Rey P, Martinelli G, Petit JY, et al. (2005) Immediate breast reconstruction and high-dose chemotherapy. Ann Plast Surg 55:250–4

Ring A, Webb A, Ashley S, et al. (2003) Is surgery necessary after complete clinical remission following neoadjuvant chemotherapy for early breast cancer? J Clin Oncol 21:4540–5

Ringberg A, Tengrup I, Aspegren K, et al. (1999) Immediate breast reconstruction after mastectomy for cancer. Eur J Surg Oncol 25:470–6

Romond EH, Perez EA, Bryant J, et al. (2005) Trastuzumab plus adjuvant chemotherapy for operable HER2-positive breast cancer. N Engl J Med 353:1673–84

Roth RS, Lowery JC, Davis J, et al. (2005) Quality of life and affective distress in women seeking immediate versus delayed breast reconstruction after mastectomy for breast cancer. Plast Reconstr Surg 116:993–1002

Roth RS, Lowery JC, Davis J, Wilkins EG (2007) Psychological factors predict patient satisfaction with postmastectomy breast reconstruction. Plast Reconstr Surg 119:2008–15

Rowland JH, Desmond KA, Meyerowitz BE, et al. (2000) Role of breast reconstructive surgery in physical and emotional outcomes among breast cancer survivors. J Natl Cancer Instit 92:1422–9

Saulis AS, Mustoe TA, Fine NA (2007) A retrospective analysis of patient satisfaction with immediate postmastectomy breast reconstruction: comparison of three common procedures. Plast Reconstr Surg 119:1669–76 ; discussion 1677–8

Schover LR (2004) Myth-busters: telling the true story of breast cancer survivorship. J Natl Cancer Inst 96:1800–1

Sepucha K, Ozanne E, Silvia K, et al. (2007) An approach to measuring the quality of breast cancer decisions. Patient Educ Couns 65:261–9

Shannon C, Ashley S, Smith IE (2003) Does timing of adjuvant chemotherapy for early breast cancer influence survival? J Clin Oncol 21:3792–7

Smith I, Procter M, Gelber RD, et al. (2007) Two-year follow-up of trastuzumab after adjuvant chemotherapy in HER2-positive breast cancer: a randomised controlled trial. Lancet 369:29–36

Tagliabue E, Agresti R, Carcangiu ML, et al. (2003) Role of HER2 in wound-induced breast carcinoma proliferation. Lancet 362:527–33

Taylor CW, Kumar S (2005) The effect of immediate breast reconstruction on adjuvant chemotherapy. Breast 14:18–21

Taylor CW, Horgan K, Dodwell D (2005) Oncological aspects of breast reconstruction. Breast 14:118–30

Wolf L (2004) The information needs of women who have undergone breast reconstruction. Part I: decision-making and sources of information. Eur J Oncol Nurs 8:211–23

Wilkins EG, Cederna PS, Lowery JC, et al. (2000) Prospective analysis of psychosocial outcomes in breast reconstruction: one-year postoperative results from the Michigan Breast Reconstruction Outcome Study. Plast Reconstr Surg 106:1014–25

Wilson CR, Brown IM, Weiller-Mithoff E, et al. (2004) Immediate breast reconstruction does not lead to a delay in the delivery of adjuvant chemotherapy. Eur J Surg Oncol 30:624–7

Yule GJ, Concannon MJ, Croll G, et al. (1996) Is there liability with chemotherapy following immediate breast construction? Plast Reconstr Surg 97:969–73

Prophylactic Mastectomy and BRCA1 or BRCA2 Gene Mutations

10

When, within a family, there are several members with cancers of the breast or ovary a genetic predisposition (GP) to these cancers should be considered. Faced with a suggestive family history (Table 10.1), an oncogenetic consultation must be offered. This may confirm a constitutional mutation to the BRCA1 and BRCA2 genes within that family.

Mutation identified in a woman, termed the "index" case, becomes the basis for testing the whole family. Even though the initial test takes a long time (several months) and may be difficult, further investigations are simplified once a target has been identified in the index case. If no mutation is identified in the relatives, they may be reassured. On the other hand, if mutation is present, the latter are at high risk of developing breast and ovarian cancer. A meta-analysis of 22 population studies summarised the risks as shown in Tables 10.2 and 10.3.

What management of the breast can be suggested to women with a GP today? We consider first prophylactic mastectomy, and then the different strategies available, according to whether the particular woman has a diagnosed breast cancer or not (see also Chapter 8).

Prophylactic Mastectomy: Principles and Efficacy of Prevention

Prophylactic mastectomy (PM) consists of removal of the mammary gland, nipple and areola and is generally accompanied by immediate breast reconstruction.

The principle behind this strategy is based on the hypothesis that breast ablation, if carried out sufficiently early in life, significantly reduces the risk of breast cancer.

Early PMs were performed in "high risk" women due to a suspicious breast cancer family history, prior to the availability of molecular diagnosis (Hartmann et al. 1999, 2001; Meijers-Heijboer et al. 2001; Rebbeck et al. 2004).

Table 10.1 Situations in which a familial genetic inquiry may be suggested generally (commencing with the affected person)

1. At least three cases of breast or ovarian cancer appearing in the same parental branch and occurring in first- or second-degree relatives
2. Two cases of breast cancer in first-degree relatives where the age of diagnosis is 40 years or below
3. Two cases of breast cancer in first-degree relatives where at least one case is male
4. Two cases in first-degree relatives with at least one case of ovarian cancer
5. The association of breast cancer with primary ovarian cancer

Table 10.2 Breast cancer risk with mutations*

	BRCA1 (%)	BRCA2 (%)
Cumulative risk to 50 years	38 (30–50)	16 (11–21)
Cumulative risk to 70 years	65 (51–75)	45 (33–54)

*95% confidence interval

Table 10.3 Ovarian cancer risk with mutations*

	BRCA1 (%)	BRCA2 (%)
Cumulative risk to 50 years	13 (8–18)	1 (0–3)
Cumulative risk to 70 years	39 (22–51)	11 (4–18)

*95% confidence interval

A recent literature review (Bermejo-Perez et al. 2007) concluded that there was a reduction in the risk of breast cancer after PM of 91–100% with a 3–7-year follow up. This limited follow up is as yet insufficient to draw any conclusions about the effect of PM on mortality.

Balancing the preventive efficacy of PM, are risks from both anaesthesia and surgery (haematoma, infection, implant-related problems and subsequent interventions) about which the patients must be carefully informed.

Several studies evaluated the social and psychological consequences of PM (Stefanek et al. 1995; Borgen et al. 1998; Frost et al. 2000; Hatcher et al. 2001; van Oostrom et al. 2003; Metcalfe et al. 2004a; Bresser et al. 2006) and concluded that satisfaction with the prophylaxis must be dissociated from satisfaction with the reconstruction itself (which depends specifically on complications and aesthetic outcomes).

Although the majority of women report a clear reduction in anxiety levels after intervention, the long-term adverse consequences, particularly sexuality (loss of erogenous sensibility secondary to nipple–areola complex ablation, body image and reactions of partners), must not be underestimated.

Management of Women Carrying BRCA1/2 Mutations Without Cancer

Two main strategies of management are currently proposed:

- MRI surveillance
- Preventative surgical or medical methods

The first strategy comprises attentive screening in order to detect small cancers that are potentially curable with early diagnosis. The American Cancer Society recently recommended that mammography be supplemented with MRI in those electing for surveillance (Saslow et al. 2007). Several prospective studies of MRI in high-risk women showed a significantly improved sensitivity (between 71 and 100%) over mammography alone (Kriege et al. 2004; Kuhl et al. 2005; MARIBS 2005; Lehman et al. 2005; Warner et al. 2004) and a lower rate of interval cancers (10% vs. 50%), although with a lower specificity. The recall rate for supplementary imaging varied between 8 and 17%, and biopsy between 3 and 15%.

The second strategy relies on prevention. The choice of a prophylactic mastectomy may only be considered if the woman concerned is completely informed of the options and associated risks. In genetically predisposed women, a prophylactic oophorectomy is recommended in order to prevent the development of ovarian cancer. In addition to the considerable reduction (of the order of 95%) of ovarian cancer risk (Rebbeck et al. 2002), there is also a reduction in breast cancer risk of approximately 50% (Rebbeck et al. 2002). Acceptance with this strategy in young women is, however, often poor.

Regarding chemoprevention, there are several arguments suggesting that tumourigenesis in these GP women is, at least initially, responsive to oestrogens and anti-oestrogens (Pujol et al. 2004) even if the majority of cancers occurring in mutated cases are not hormone-receptor positive. To date, several anti-oestrogens have been tested in women at risk of breast cancer: tamoxifen (Fisher et al. 2005; Cuzick et al. 2003, 2007; Powles et al. 2007), raloxifen (Vogel et al. 2006) and anti-aromatases.

In France, these compounds are neither licensed for this condition nor can they be used in clinical trials.

The management of mammary risk in GP women has been the subject of two collective reports (Eisinger et al. 1998, 2004), and it is based on these that the Institut Curie offers patients carrying either a mutation or a suggestive family history the specific therapeutic pathway. In addition to the geneticist, all patients are routinely offered consultations with a gynaecologist, psychologist, and an oncoplastic surgeon.

The final decision is made after multidisciplinary discussion with all parties.

Importantly, the advice and participation of the partner in any decision is recommended as is a delay of at least four months for reflection.

Diagnosis of a Breast Cancer in a Woman with BRCA1/2 Mutation

When a primary breast cancer is diagnosed during surveillance of a GP woman, the therapeutic strategy must take account of the gene mutation.

The prognosis of tumours occurring in the context of BRCA1 or BRCA2 remains the source of discussion: poor according to some (Stoppa-Lyonnet et al. 2000), and no different according to others (Bonadona et al. 2007; Brekelmans et al. 2007).

On the other hand, it is well established that the risk of contralateral breast cancer is increased: of the order of 2–3% per annum with BRCA2 and 3–4% for BRCA1 (Metcalfe et al. 2004b), compared to 0.7% for the population in general.

In breast cancer amenable to conservative treatment, two options may be discussed: either conservative treatment, for which we aim as standard, or nonconservative treatment; the latter involving delayed breast reconstruction, after adjuvant chemotherapy and/or radiotherapy, which may be combined with contralateral prophylactic mastectomy and immediate reconstruction to reduce the risk of contralateral tumour development (Vansprundel et al. 2005).

Discovery of BRCA1/2 Mutation After Diagnosis of Breast Cancer

BRCA1/2 mutation may also be diagnosed in a woman already treated for breast cancer.

In the case of mastectomy, one may offer at the time of any secondary surgery, a contralateral prophylactic mastectomy with IBR. Another option is surveillance of the contralateral breast with MRI.

If the initial treatment is conservative, the discussion is more delicate. In fact, it appears that the risk of ipsilateral recurrence will be no different to that of anyone else with cancer in the following ten years (Kirova et al. 2005; Pierce et al. 2006), which suggests a protective effect of irradiation. The increased risk of contralateral cancer, however, remains.

Women who do not wish to risk a second cancer may thus opt for a contralateral PM with IBR, or even for bilateral mastectomy, considering the potential problems involved in reconstructing an already irradiated breast.

High Family Risk Without Identified Mutation

Even with a high familial incidence of breast cancer, BRCA1/2 mutation is sometimes not identified genetically and statistical methods of predicting tumour risk

may be used instead (Eisinger et al. 2004). These differ between teams. In an unaffected woman, or one presenting with breast cancer, a request for PM may be considered whilst awaiting validation, taking note of the family history. This indication for PM will only therefore be accepted in the setting of a multidisciplinary decision.

Conclusion

In conclusion, the management of breast and ovarian risk in GP is delicate. It is currently only possible in a specialist environment. Certain questions—such as the management of breast cancer in a GP woman, or the strategy suggested to a woman who has been already treated in a conservative fashion—remain sources of discussion, and require prospective research.

References

Bermejo-Pérez M, Marquez-Calderon S, Llanos-Méndes A (2007) Effectiveness of preventive interventions in *BRCA1/2* gene mutation carriers: a systematic review. Int J Cancer 121:225–31

Bonadona V, Dussart-Moser S, Voirin N, et al. (2007) Prognosis of early-onset breast cancer based on BRCA1/2 mutation status in a French population-based cohort and review. Breast Cancer Res Treat 101(2):233–45

Borgen PI, Hill AD, Tran KN, et al. (1998) Patient regrets after bilateral prophylactic mastectomy. Ann Surg Oncol 5(7):603–6

Brekelmans CT, Tilanus-Linthorst MM, Seynaeve C, et al. (2007) Tumour characteristics, survival and prognostic factors of hereditary breast cancer from BRCA2-, BRCA1- and non-BRCA1/2 families as compared to sporadic breast cancer cases. Eur J Cancer 43(5):867–76

Bresser P, Seynaeve C, Vangool A, et al. (2006) Satisfaction with prophylactic mastectomy and breast reconstruction in genetically predisposed women. Plast Reconstr Surg 117:1675–82

Cuzick J, Powles T, Veronesi U, et al. (2003) Overview of the main outcomes in breast-cancer prevention trials. Lancet 361(9354):296–300

Cuzick J, Forbes J, Sestak I, et al. (2007) Long-term results of tamoxifen prophylaxis for breast cancer—96 month follow-up of the randomized IBIS-I trial. J Natl Cancer Inst 99:272–82

Eisinger F, Alby N, Bremond A, et al. (1998) INSERM-FNCLCC Collective Expert's Report. Recommendations for management of women having a genetic risk of developing breast and/or ovarian cancer. National Federation of Centers of the Fight Against Cancer. Ann Endocrinol 59(6):470–84

Eisinger F, Bressac B, Castaigne D, et al. (2004) Identification et prise en charge des prédispositions héréditaires aux cancers du sein et de l'ovaire (mise à jour 2004). Bull Cancer 91(3):219–37

Fisher B, Costantino J, Wickerham D, et al. (2005) Tamoxifen for the prevention of breast cancer: current status of the national surgical adjuvant breast and bowel project P1-Study. J Natl Cancer Inst 97:1652–62

Frost MH, Schaid DJ, Sellers TA, et al. (2000) Long-term satisfaction and psychological and social function following bilateral prophylactic mastectomy. JAMA 284(3):319–24

Hartmann LC, Schaid DJ, Woods JE, et al. (1999) Efficacy of bilateral prophylactic mastectomy in women with a family history of breast cancer. N Engl J Med 340(2):77–84

Hartmann LC, Sellers TA, Schaid DJ, et al. (2001) Efficacy of bilateral prophylactic mastectomy in BRCA1 and BRCA2 gene mutation carriers. J Natl Cancer Inst 93(21):1633–7

Hatcher MB, Fallowfield L, A'Hern R (2001) The psychosocial impact of bilateral prophylactic mastectomy: prospective study using questionnaires and semistructured interviews. BMJ 322(7278):76

Kirova YM, Stoppa-Lyonnet D, Savignoni A, et al. (2005). Risk of breast cancer recurrence and contralateral breast cancer in relation to BRCA1 and BRCA2 mutation status following breast-conserving surgery and radiotherapy. Eur J Cancer 41(15):2304–11

Kriege M, Brekelmans C, Boetes C, et al. (2004) Efficacy of MRI and mammography for breast-cancer screening in women with a familial or genetic predisposition. N Engl J Med 351(5):427–37

Kuhl C, Schrading S, Leutner C, et al. (2005) Mammography, breast ultrasound, and magnetic resonance imaging for surveillance of women at high familial risk of breast cancer. J Clin Oncol 23(33):8469–76

Lehman C, Blume J, Weatherall P, et al. (2005) Screening women at high risk for breast cancer with mammography and magnetic resonance imaging. Cancer 103:1898–905

MARIBS Study Group (2005) Screening with magnetic resonance imaging and mammography of a UK population at high familial risk of breast cancer: a prospective multicentre cohort study (MARIBS). Lancet 365:1769–78

Meijers-Heijboer H, van Geel B, van Putten WL, et al. (2001) Breast cancer after prophylactic bilateral mastectomy in women with a BRCA1 or BRCA2 mutation. N Engl J Med 345(3):159–64

Metcalfe K, Esplen M, Goel V, et al. (2004a) Psychosocial functioning in women who have undergone bilateral prophylactic mastectomy. Psychooncology 13:14–25

Metcalfe K, Lynch HT, Ghadirian P, Tung N, et al. (2004b) Contralateral breast cancer in BRCA1 and BRCA2 mutation carriers. J Clin Oncol 22(12):2328–35

Pierce LJ, Levin AM, Rebbeck TR, et al. (2006) Ten-year multi-institutional results of breast-conserving surgery and radiotherapy in BRCA1/2-associated stage I/II breast cancer. J Clin Oncol 24(16):2437–43

Powles T, Ashley S, Tidy A, et al. (2007) Twenty-year follow-up of the Royal Marsden randomized, double-blinded tamoxifen breast cancer prevention trial. J Natl Cancer Inst 99:283–90

Pujol P, This P, Noruzinia M, et al. (2004) Estrogens, antiestrogens and familial breast cancer. Bull Cancer 91(7–8):583–91

Rebbeck T, Lynch H, Neuhausen S (2002) Prophylactic oophorectomy in carriers of BRCA1 or BRCA2 mutations. N Engl J Med 346:1616–22

Rebbeck T, Friebel T, Lynch H, et al. (2004) Bilateral prophylactic mastectomy reduces breast cancer risk in BRCA1 and BRCA2 mutations carriers: the PROSE study group. J Clin Oncol 22(6):1055–62

Saslow D, Boetes C, Burke W, et al. (2007) American Cancer Society Guidelines for breast screening with MRI as an adjunct to mammography. CA Cancer J Clin 57:75–89

Stefanek M, Helzlsouer KJ, Wilcox P, et al. (1995) Predictors of and satisfaction with bilateral prophylactic mastectomy. Prev Med 24:412–9

Stoppa-Lyonnet D, Ansquer Y, Dreyfus H, et al. (2000) Familial invasive breast cancers: worse outcome related to BRCA1 mutations. J Clin Oncol 18(24):4053–9

van Oostrom I, Meijers Heijboer H, Lodder L, et al. (2003) Long-term psychological impact of carrying a BRCA1/2 mutation and prophylactic surgery: a 5 year follow-up study. J Clin Oncol 21:3867–74

Vansprundel T, Schmidt M, Rookus M, et al. (2005) Risk reduction of controlateral breast cancer and survival after contralateral prophylactic mastectomy in BRCA1 or BRCA2 mutation carriers. Br J Cancer 93:287–92

Vogel V, Costantino J, Wickerham D, et al. (2006) Effects of tamoxifen vs raloxifene on the risk of developing invasive breast cancer and other disease outcomes: The NSABP study of Tamoxifen and Raloxifen (STAR) P2 trial. JAMA 295:2727–41

Warner E, Plewes D, Hill K, et al. (2004) Surveillance of BRCA1 and BRCA2 mutation carriers with magnetic resonance imaging, ultrasound, mammography, and clinical breast examination. JAMA 292:1317–25

Glossary

AAF	Abdominal advancement flap
ACC	Adverse capsular contracture
BCT	Breast-conserving therapy
BRCA	BReast CAncer gene
CT	Computed tomography
DIEA	Deep inferior epigastric artery
DIEP	Deep inferior epigastric perforator (flap)
GP	Genetic predisposition
IBR/DBR	Immediate/delayed breast reconstruction
IMF	Inframammary fold
LD (ALD)	Latissimus dorsi (autologous LD)
MDT	Multidisciplinary team
MRI	Magnetic resonance imaging
NAC	Nipple–areolar complex
OBS	Oncoplastic breast surgery
PM	Prophylactic mastectomy
SIEA	Superficial inferior epigastric artery
SNB/SLNB	Sentinel node/sentinel lymph node biopsy
TRAM	Transverse rectus abdominis musculocutaneous (flap)

Index